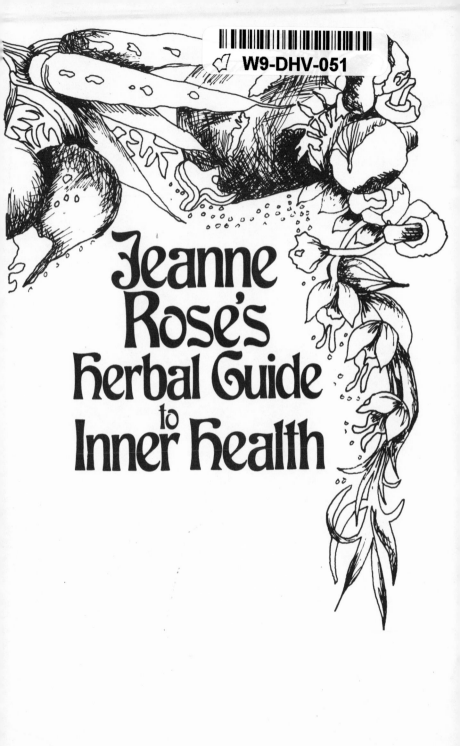

Jeanne Rose's Herbal Guide to Inner Health

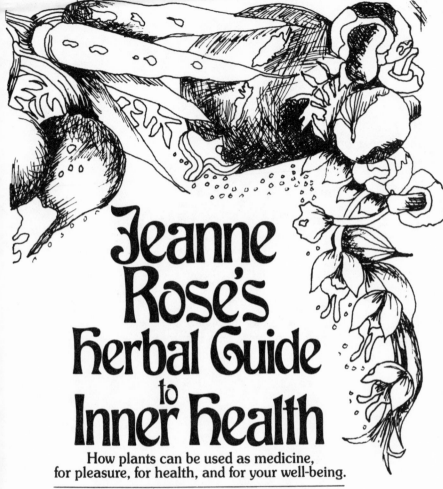

Jeanne Rose's Herbal Guide to Inner Health

How plants can be used as medicine,
for pleasure, for health, and for your well-being.

Illustrated by Michael S. Moore
with John Hulburd

GROSSET & DUNLAP
A FILMWAYS COMPANY
Publishers • New York

Other Books by Jeanne Rose

Herbs & Things

Jeanne Rose's Herbal Body Book:
The Herbal Way to Natural Beauty and Health
for Men and Women

Kitchen Cosmetics

*"My Majesty made for him a garden
anew in order to present to him
vegetables and all beautiful flowers."*

—Offerings of Thutmose III
to Amon-Ra
(1500 B.C.)

Dedication

to john who put into motion such changes

to jimmy who said,
*"changes are like
little black flowers
that open
slowly in the dark"*

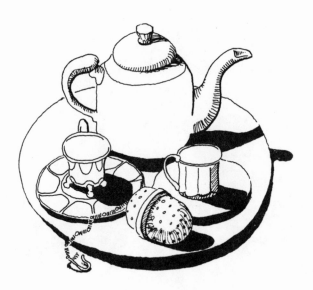

Acknowledgments

"You have such beautiful hair"—December 10, 1976—"Will you ride the rails with me to Jackson Hole, Wyoming, this summer?" —I didn't—but it was a nice idea.

To the people who by their efforts give me the time to do the work I most enjoy, and that is, playing with plants: Joyce, Tom, H. Ron, my personal editor Jennifer, my Grosset editor Joyce, to Pam and to Helen Gannaway.

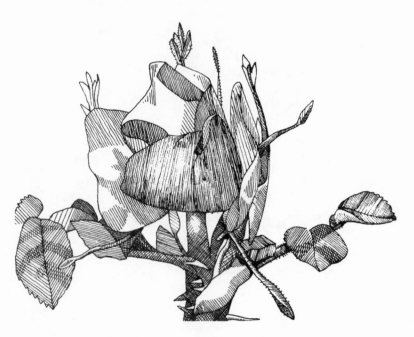

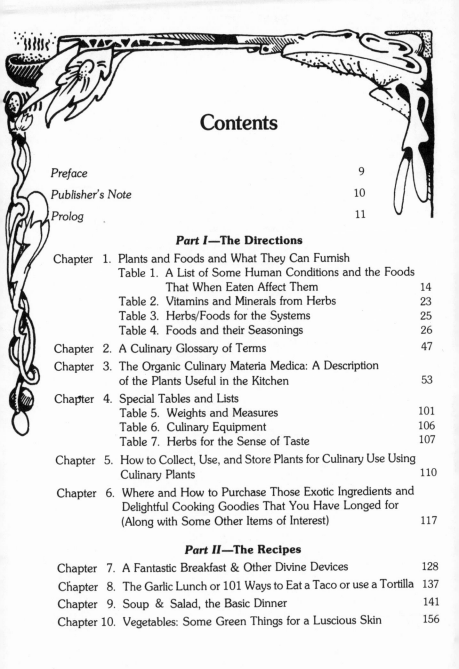

Contents

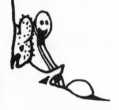

Part III—The Secrets

Preface

I think it is a little presumptuous of me to be writing a cookbook. I rarely cook complicated or exotic foods. I am interested in food more as nourishment to the spirit and less as a means of fattening up an individual. Let food be your medicine. Cook wholesome, simple things that are pleasant to look at and fulfilling to the taste. Save the sensuously wicked sauces and complicated cooking of *haute cuisine* for the expert, and, if you really must enjoy these devilish delights, go out to dinner once in a while.

When my publishers asked me to write a cookbook, my first reaction was one of disbelief. I didn't think that I knew a hundred recipes. I asked my family at one of our infrequent discussions to list everything I make that they really like to eat. We were all surprised to find out that I had hundreds of frequently used recipes. My recipes are not original. They come from my French mother, my Spanish father, my American Indian forebear, and my various in-laws. These recipes have been used by me and my family many times. We no longer use exact ingredients or recipes but change ingredients and recipes to suit the time and season of the year.

As in all my books, it is not the recipes themselves that are truly important but the information surrounding them that counts. I do hope you will experiment using whatever fresh herbs or dried herbs you have at hand. Be generous with your use of herbs and stingy with your use of salt. Soon you will become familiar with the taste of the real food without salt, and you will come to like food more and the salt taste less.

Have fun—and good cooking.

Jeanne Rose
Spring 1979

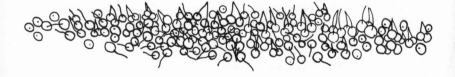

9

Moderation in all things is all that counts

—Jeanne Rose,
The Herbal Body Book

Publisher's Note

All plants, like all medicines, may be dangerous, particularly to those subject to allergic reactions, if used improperly—if they are taken internally when prescribed for external use, if they are taken in excess or immoderately, or if they are taken for too long a time. Allergic reactions and unpredictable sensitivities may develop. There are other factors to consider as well: since the strength of wild herbs varies, knowledge of their growing conditions is helpful. Be sure your herbs are fresh and keep conditions of use as sterile as possible.

We do not advocate, endorse, or guarantee the curative effects of any of the substances listed in this book. We have made every effort to see that any botanical that is dangerous or potentially dangerous has been noted as such. When you use herbs, recognize their potency and use them with care. Medical consultation is recommended for those recipes that might be marked as dangerous.

The botanical names listed after each herb do not always refer to one species only, but also to others, which in herbal medicine have been recognized as substitutes.

Prolog

My friend Erica introduced me to her vision of perfect health. It is a picture she keeps in her mind all the time, and when things get rough she drags out that vision and looks at it for awhile and then things get better. That vision of hers got me thinking about my own picture/vision of perfect health. I thought about it for awhile and one day there it was full consciousness in front of me.

My skin all over lightly green, a spring green, mottled with lovely patches of purple, sort of a pattern of paisley. I have short, strong wings, rather leathery in texture; they are pink. My skin is tight feeling, somewhat glabrous, and comfortable on me. I skim lightly over the ground, my rootlets barely touching the brown earth, and orbs of flashing light dance around.

I find this picture to be an aid in keeping myself healthy. Why? It gives me a good feeling, a rather bizarre but comfortable feeling, a meditation that I can concentrate upon nightly before sleep—it chases all the nerves away, the upset, the virus trying to sneak up on me, the bacteria trying to gét a hold—I just lift up and fly away.

Why don't you sit down some day and meditate your way to your own picture of health? How exactly does it feel and what exactly does it look like to you? Dream your dreams on a mugwort and rosebud pillow, eat eight-jewel rice and maybe you too will be healthier and happier because of your vision.

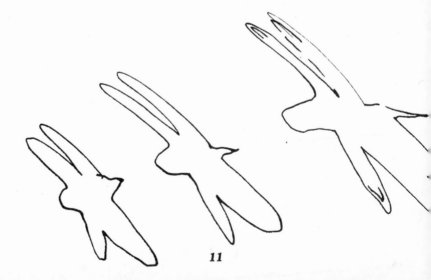

11

HERBS & SIMPLES

"My Aunt Gudrun . . . knew a great deal about herbs and simples, though
I used to think she made her potions more noxious than need be.
"And she would watch the sick one swallow it with such a look as if to
say, 'I'll learn ye to be took sick.' "

— Mary Webb, *Armour Wherein He Trusted*

I suppose you could make medicines that would be distasteful but it seems ever so
much better to let your kitchen become your apothecary. Make foods the carrier of
health and if you happen to get sick, then let foods become your medicine.

Part I
The Directions

Let thy kitchen be thy apothecary
and
Let foods be your medicine

Hippocratus

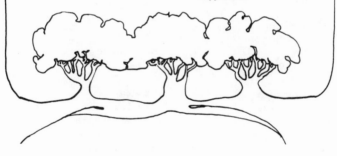

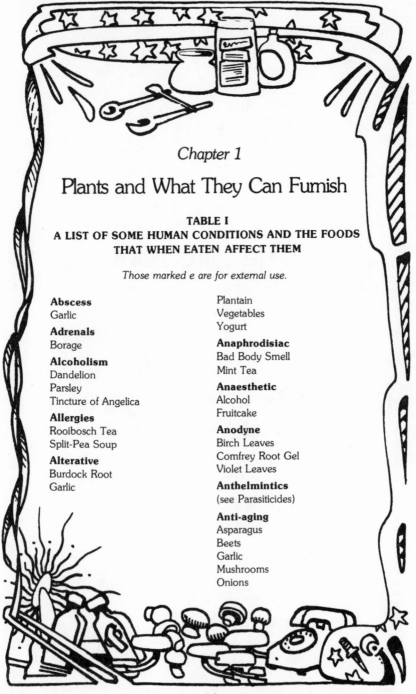

Chapter 1

Plants and What They Can Furnish

TABLE I
**A LIST OF SOME HUMAN CONDITIONS AND THE FOODS
THAT WHEN EATEN AFFECT THEM**

Those marked e are for external use.

Abscess
Garlic

Adrenals
Borage

Alcoholism
Dandelion
Parsley
Tincture of Angelica

Allergies
Rooibosch Tea
Split-Pea Soup

Alterative
Burdock Root
Garlic

Plantain
Vegetables
Yogurt

Anaphrodisiac
Bad Body Smell
Mint Tea

Anaesthetic
Alcohol
Fruitcake

Anodyne
Birch Leaves
Comfrey Root Gel
Violet Leaves

Anthelmintics
(see Parasiticides)

Anti-aging
Asparagus
Beets
Garlic
Mushrooms
Onions

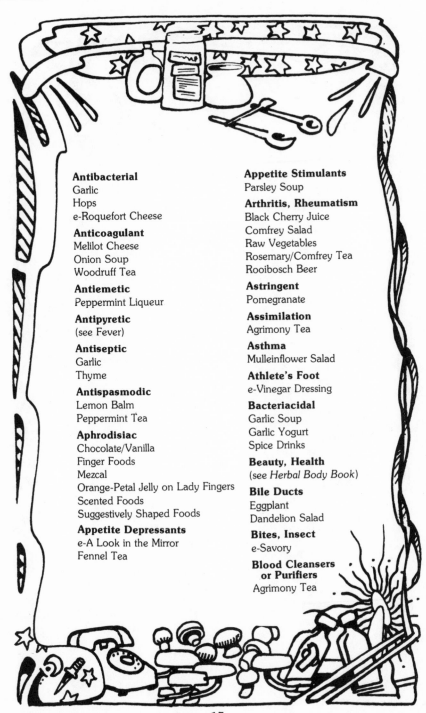

Antibacterial
Garlic
Hops
e-Roquefort Cheese

Anticoagulant
Melilot Cheese
Onion Soup
Woodruff Tea

Antiemetic
Peppermint Liqueur

Antipyretic
(see Fever)

Antiseptic
Garlic
Thyme

Antispasmodic
Lemon Balm
Peppermint Tea

Aphrodisiac
Chocolate/Vanilla
Finger Foods
Mezcal
Orange-Petal Jelly on Lady Fingers
Scented Foods
Suggestively Shaped Foods

Appetite Depressants
e-A Look in the Mirror
Fennel Tea

Appetite Stimulants
Parsley Soup

Arthritis, Rheumatism
Black Cherry Juice
Comfrey Salad
Raw Vegetables
Rosemary/Comfrey Tea
Rooibosch Beer

Astringent
Pomegranate

Assimilation
Agrimony Tea

Asthma
Mulleinflower Salad

Athlete's Foot
e-Vinegar Dressing

Bacteriacidal
Garlic Soup
Garlic Yogurt
Spice Drinks

Beauty, Health
(see *Herbal Body Book*)

Bile Ducts
Eggplant
Dandelion Salad

Bites, Insect
e-Savory

**Blood Cleansers
   or Purifiers**
Agrimony Tea

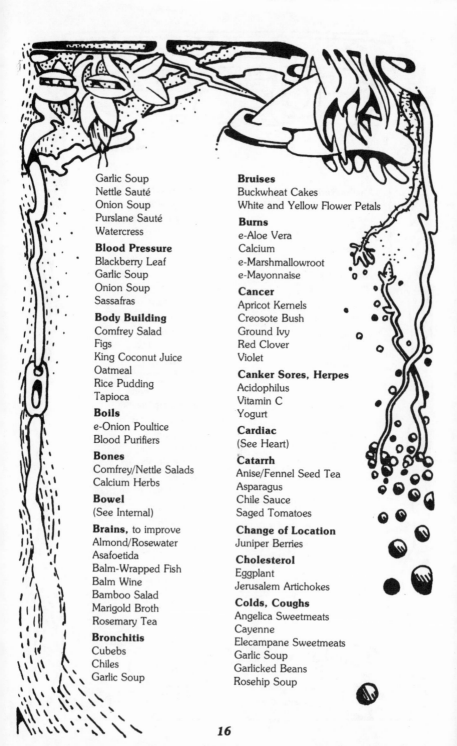

Garlic Soup
Nettle Sauté
Onion Soup
Purslane Sauté
Watercress

Blood Pressure
Blackberry Leaf
Garlic Soup
Onion Soup
Sassafras

Body Building
Comfrey Salad
Figs
King Coconut Juice
Oatmeal
Rice Pudding
Tapioca

Boils
e-Onion Poultice
Blood Purifiers

Bones
Comfrey/Nettle Salads
Calcium Herbs

Bowel
(See Internal)

Brains, to improve
Almond/Rosewater
Asafoetida
Balm-Wrapped Fish
Balm Wine
Bamboo Salad
Marigold Broth
Rosemary Tea

Bronchitis
Cubebs
Chiles
Garlic Soup

Bruises
Buckwheat Cakes
White and Yellow Flower Petals

Burns
e-Aloe Vera
Calcium
e-Marshmallowroot
e-Mayonnaise

Cancer
Apricot Kernels
Creosote Bush
Ground Ivy
Red Clover
Violet

Canker Sores, Herpes
Acidophilus
Vitamin C
Yogurt

Cardiac
(See Heart)

Catarrh
Anise/Fennel Seed Tea
Asparagus
Chile Sauce
Saged Tomatoes

Change of Location
Juniper Berries

Cholesterol
Eggplant
Jerusalem Artichokes

Colds, Coughs
Angelica Sweetmeats
Cayenne
Elecampane Sweetmeats
Garlic Soup
Garlicked Beans
Rosehip Soup

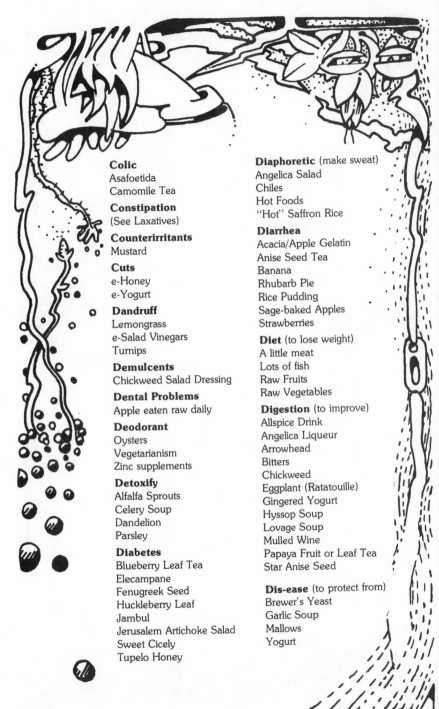

Colic
Asafoetida
Camomile Tea

Constipation
(See Laxatives)

Counterirritants
Mustard

Cuts
e-Honey
e-Yogurt

Dandruff
Lemongrass
e-Salad Vinegars
Turnips

Demulcents
Chickweed Salad Dressing

Dental Problems
Apple eaten raw daily

Deodorant
Oysters
Vegetarianism
Zinc supplements

Detoxify
Alfalfa Sprouts
Celery Soup
Dandelion
Parsley

Diabetes
Blueberry Leaf Tea
Elecampane
Fenugreek Seed
Huckleberry Leaf
Jambul
Jerusalem Artichoke Salad
Sweet Cicely
Tupelo Honey

Diaphoretic (make sweat)
Angelica Salad
Chiles
Hot Foods
"Hot" Saffron Rice

Diarrhea
Acacia/Apple Gelatin
Anise Seed Tea
Banana
Rhubarb Pie
Rice Pudding
Sage-baked Apples
Strawberries

Diet (to lose weight)
A little meat
Lots of fish
Raw Fruits
Raw Vegetables

Digestion (to improve)
Allspice Drink
Angelica Liqueur
Arrowhead
Bitters
Chickweed
Eggplant (Ratatouille)
Gingered Yogurt
Hyssop Soup
Lovage Soup
Mulled Wine
Papaya Fruit or Leaf Tea
Star Anise Seed

Dis-ease (to protect from)
Brewer's Yeast
Garlic Soup
Mallows
Yogurt

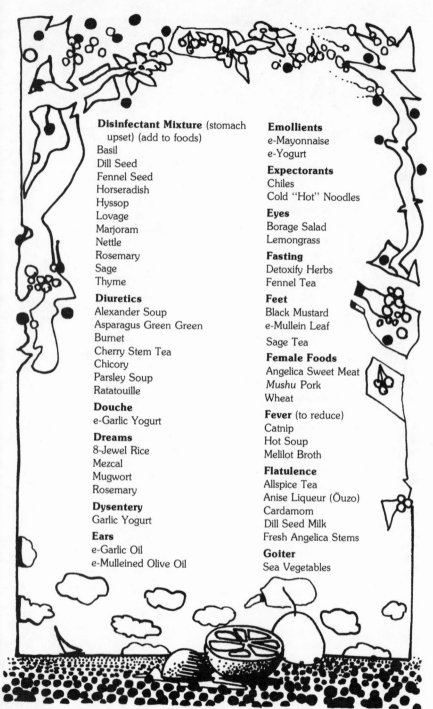

Disinfectant Mixture (stomach upset) (add to foods)
Basil
Dill Seed
Fennel Seed
Horseradish
Hyssop
Lovage
Marjoram
Nettle
Rosemary
Sage
Thyme

Diuretics
Alexander Soup
Asparagus Green Green
Burnet
Cherry Stem Tea
Chicory
Parsley Soup
Ratatouille

Douche
e-Garlic Yogurt

Dreams
8-Jewel Rice
Mezcal
Mugwort
Rosemary

Dysentery
Garlic Yogurt

Ears
e-Garlic Oil
e-Mulleined Olive Oil

Emollients
e-Mayonnaise
e-Yogurt

Expectorants
Chiles
Cold "Hot" Noodles

Eyes
Borage Salad
Lemongrass

Fasting
Detoxify Herbs
Fennel Tea

Feet
Black Mustard
e-Mullein Leaf
Sage Tea

Female Foods
Angelica Sweet Meat
Mushu Pork
Wheat

Fever (to reduce)
Catnip
Hot Soup
Melilot Broth

Flatulence
Allspice Tea
Anise Liqueur (Öuzo)
Cardamom
Dill Seed Milk
Fresh Angelica Stems

Goiter
Sea Vegetables

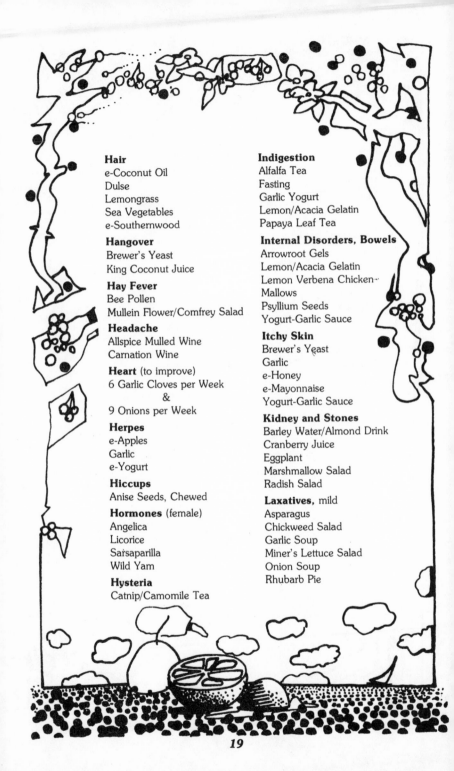

Hair
e-Coconut Oil
Dulse
Lemongrass
Sea Vegetables
e-Southernwood

Hangover
Brewer's Yeast
King Coconut Juice

Hay Fever
Bee Pollen
Mullein Flower/Comfrey Salad

Headache
Allspice Mulled Wine
Carnation Wine

Heart (to improve)
6 Garlic Cloves per Week
&
9 Onions per Week

Herpes
e-Apples
Garlic
e-Yogurt

Hiccups
Anise Seeds, Chewed

Hormones (female)
Angelica
Licorice
Sarsaparilla
Wild Yam

Hysteria
Catnip/Camomile Tea

Indigestion
Alfalfa Tea
Fasting
Garlic Yogurt
Lemon/Acacia Gelatin
Papaya Leaf Tea

Internal Disorders, Bowels
Arrowroot Gels
Lemon/Acacia Gelatin
Lemon Verbena Chicken-
Mallows
Psyllium Seeds
Yogurt-Garlic Sauce

Itchy Skin
Brewer's Yeast
Garlic
e-Honey
e-Mayonnaise
Yogurt-Garlic Sauce

Kidney and Stones
Barley Water/Almond Drink
Cranberry Juice
Eggplant
Marshmallow Salad
Radish Salad

Laxatives, mild
Asparagus
Chickweed Salad
Garlic Soup
Miner's Lettuce Salad
Onion Soup
Rhubarb Pie

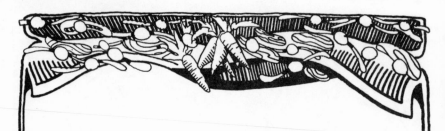

Liver
Dandelion
Eggplant
Horseradish
Hyssop
Nasturtium Salad
Sage
Santolina

Male Food
Barley

Memory
Lemon Balm
Rosemary-Stuffed Chicken
Rosemary Lemonade

Menstrual
Amaranth
Candied Angelica Roots
Clary Beer
Pennyroyal
Rue in a Salad
Sweet Cicely

Menopause
Licorice

Mental Disorders
Carnation
Marijuana Tea
Primrose
Wood Betony

Mother's Milk (to increase)
Fennel Seed Tea

Mother's Milk (to decrease)
Sage
Saged Tomatoes

Mouth, Teeth, Gums
Apples

Muscle
Linden Tisane
Sage
Wallflower

Nerves
Basil-stuffed Mushrooms
Poppy Seed

Obesity (to reduce)
Alfalfa/Dandelion Tea
Chickweed
Nettle Purée
Parsley
Potato
Samphire Salad

Parasiticides
Garlic Soup
Pomegranate Seeds
Salsa Mexicana

Poison Ivy or Oak
e-Honey
e-Yogurt

Prostate
Pumpkin Seed/Garlic Soup
Sunflower Seed

Protein
Combined Flowers & Grasses
Comfrey
Dulse
Legumes & Cereals
Nuts & Seeds

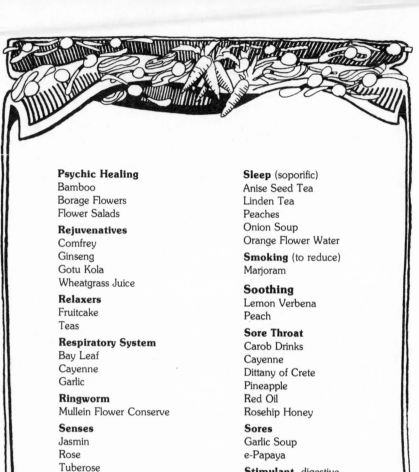

Psychic Healing
Bamboo
Borage Flowers
Flower Salads

Rejuvenatives
Comfrey
Ginseng
Gotu Kola
Wheatgrass Juice

Relaxers
Fruitcake
Teas

Respiratory System
Bay Leaf
Cayenne
Garlic

Ringworm
Mullein Flower Conserve

Senses
Jasmin
Rose
Tuberose

Sinus
Garlic Soup
Steamed Zucchini (Favorite Zucchini)

Skin
e-Almond Facials
Blender Mayonnaise
Burdock Root
Pansy
Parsley
Vegetables
Watercress

Sleep (soporific)
Anise Seed Tea
Linden Tea
Peaches
Onion Soup
Orange Flower Water

Smoking (to reduce)
Marjoram

Soothing
Lemon Verbena
Peach

Sore Throat
Carob Drinks
Cayenne
Dittany of Crete
Pineapple
Red Oil
Rosehip Honey

Sores
Garlic Soup
e-Papaya

Stimulant, digestive
Allspice Tea
Cayenne
Chocolate
Coffee
Cubebs

Stomach Ache
Acacia/Apple Gelatin
Angostura Bitters
Cabbage Soup
Chickweed Salad Dressing
Ginger Yogurt
Mulleined Milk

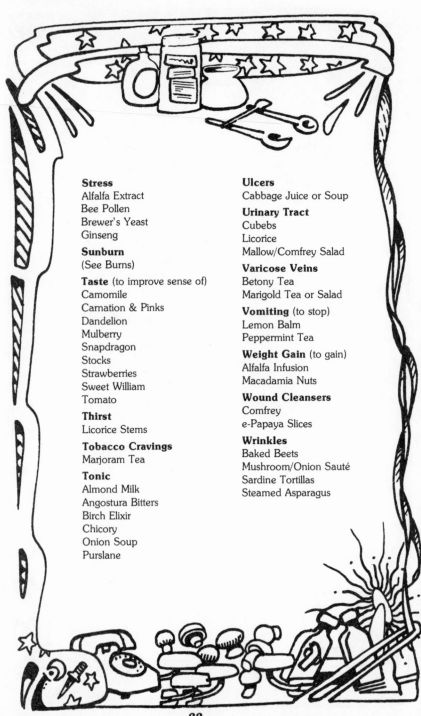

Stress
Alfalfa Extract
Bee Pollen
Brewer's Yeast
Ginseng

Sunburn
(See Burns)

Taste (to improve sense of)
Camomile
Carnation & Pinks
Dandelion
Mulberry
Snapdragon
Stocks
Strawberries
Sweet William
Tomato

Thirst
Licorice Stems

Tobacco Cravings
Marjoram Tea

Tonic
Almond Milk
Angostura Bitters
Birch Elixir
Chicory
Onion Soup
Purslane

Ulcers
Cabbage Juice or Soup

Urinary Tract
Cubebs
Licorice
Mallow/Comfrey Salad

Varicose Veins
Betony Tea
Marigold Tea or Salad

Vomiting (to stop)
Lemon Balm
Peppermint Tea

Weight Gain (to gain)
Alfalfa Infusion
Macadamia Nuts

Wound Cleansers
Comfrey
e-Papaya Slices

Wrinkles
Baked Beets
Mushroom/Onion Sauté
Sardine Tortillas
Steamed Asparagus

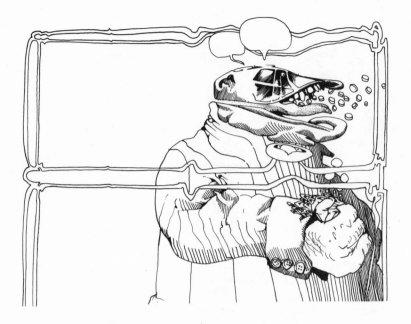

TABLE 2
VITAMINS AND MINERALS FROM HERBS

Vitamin A
Alfalfa
Annatto Seeds
Apricot
Avocado
Cayenne
Cress
Collard
Carrot
Chiles
Dandelion
Dock
Elderberries
Greens
Kale
Lamb's quarters
Lemongrass
Nettle
Okra
Parsley
Peppers
Paprika
Plantain
Violet

Vitamin B1 (Thiamine)
Dulse
Kelp
Peanut
Piñon Nut
Rice Bran
Soybean
Sunflower
Walnuts
Wheat Germ

Vitamin B2 (Riboflavin)
Almonds
Brewer's Yeast
Chiles
Dulse
Kelp
Lamb's quarters
Mushrooms
Saffron
Wheat Germ
Wild Rice

Vitamin B6 (Pyridoxine)
Beet

Blackstrap Molasses
Cabbage
Wheat Bran
Wheat Germ
Yeast

Vitamin B12
Alfalfa
Comfrey
Dulse
Fenugreek
Kelp

Vitamin C
Acerola Juice
Black Currant
Cabbage
Chiles, Greens & Red
Collard
Dock
Greens
Guava
Kale
Lemon with Peel
Nasturtium

23

Nettle
Orange with Peel
Parsley
Peppers, Sweet Red
& Green
Pine Needles
Paprika
Rosehips
Sorrel
Strawberry Leaf
Violet Leaf
Watercress

Vitamin D
Avocado
Milk
Watercress
Wheat Germ

Vitamin E
Alfalfa
Avocado
Dandelion
Pumpkin Seeds
Sesame Seeds
Sunflower Seeds
Wheat Germ

Vitamin G
Bananas
Greens

Vitamin K (coagulant)
Alfalfa
Chestnuts
Shepherd's-purse

MINERALS

Bioflavonoids
Apricot
Buckwheat
Citrus Peels
Parsley
Yellow & White Flower Petals

Calcium
Borage
Chickweed
Comfrey
Dandelion

Chlorine
Avocado

Copper
Chickweed

Iron
Arrach
Borage
Chenopodiaceae
Chickweed
Comfrey
Good-King-Henry
Nettle

Manganese
Beet
Carrot
Celery
Chives
Cucumber
Parsley

Potassium
Avocado
Banana
Borage
Dandelion
Potato

Protein
Flowers & Grasses
Nuts & Seeds

Sulfur
Avocado
Dandelion
Garlic
Onion
Watercress

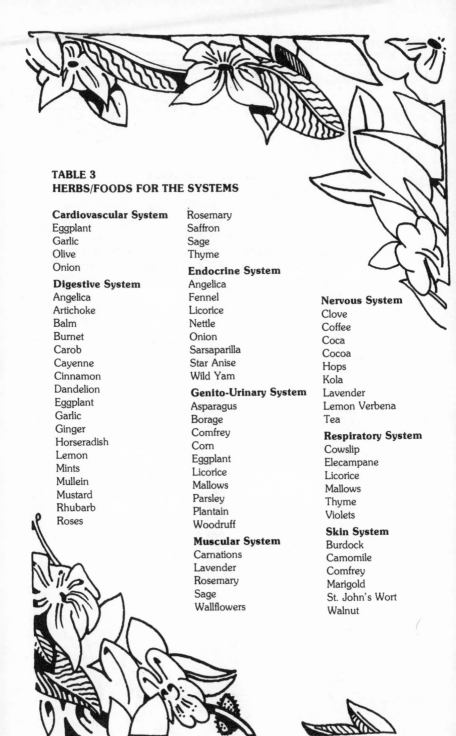

TABLE 3
HERBS/FOODS FOR THE SYSTEMS

Cardiovascular System
Eggplant
Garlic
Olive
Onion

Digestive System
Angelica
Artichoke
Balm
Burnet
Carob
Cayenne
Cinnamon
Dandelion
Eggplant
Garlic
Ginger
Horseradish
Lemon
Mints
Mullein
Mustard
Rhubarb
Roses

Rosemary
Saffron
Sage
Thyme

Endocrine System
Angelica
Fennel
Licorice
Nettle
Onion
Sarsaparilla
Star Anise
Wild Yam

Genito-Urinary System
Asparagus
Borage
Comfrey
Corn
Eggplant
Licorice
Mallows
Parsley
Plantain
Woodruff

Muscular System
Carnations
Lavender
Rosemary
Sage
Wallflowers

Nervous System
Clove
Coffee
Coca
Cocoa
Hops
Kola
Lavender
Lemon Verbena
Tea

Respiratory System
Cowslip
Elecampane
Licorice
Mallows
Thyme
Violets

Skin System
Burdock
Camomile
Comfrey
Marigold
St. John's Wort
Walnut

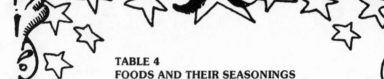

TABLE 4
FOODS AND THEIR SEASONINGS

Having always wanted to know which seasoning herbs went with which foods rather than the other way 'round, I found that I had to make my own list. Most lists showed an herb, like Basil, and then proceeded to list several things that went with it. This seemed rather backwards to me. I hope that the list I have compiled will help you to use herbs and seasoning spices more often. The list is certainly not complete but it is a good beginning.

Abalone
Capers
Chives
Garlic
Lemon
Parsley
Shallots

Acorn Squash
Allspice
Basil
Cinnamon
Nutmeg
Rosemary

Anchovy
Lemon Juice
Parsley
Pepper
Rosemary
Tomato

Applesauce
Allspice
Cinnamon
Lemon
Mace
Nutmeg
Red Currant
Vanilla

Apricots
Ginger
Lemon Rind
Mace
Nutmeg

Artichokes
Bay
Celery
Garlic
Lovage
Nasturtium Seedpods
Oregano
Thyme

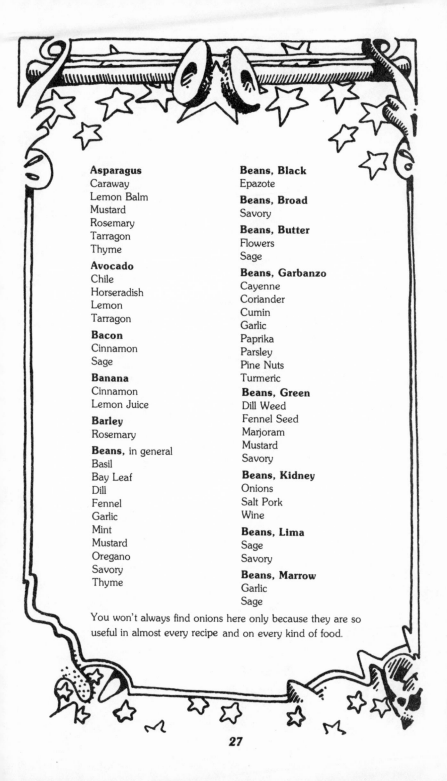

Asparagus
Caraway
Lemon Balm
Mustard
Rosemary
Tarragon
Thyme

Avocado
Chile
Horseradish
Lemon
Tarragon

Bacon
Cinnamon
Sage

Banana
Cinnamon
Lemon Juice

Barley
Rosemary

Beans, in general
Basil
Bay Leaf
Dill
Fennel
Garlic
Mint
Mustard
Oregano
Savory
Thyme

Beans, Black
Epazote

Beans, Broad
Savory

Beans, Butter
Flowers
Sage

Beans, Garbanzo
Cayenne
Coriander
Cumin
Garlic
Paprika
Parsley
Pine Nuts
Turmeric

Beans, Green
Dill Weed
Fennel Seed
Marjoram
Mustard
Savory

Beans, Kidney
Onions
Salt Pork
Wine

Beans, Lima
Sage
Savory

Beans, Marrow
Garlic
Sage

You won't always find onions here only because they are so useful in almost every recipe and on every kind of food.

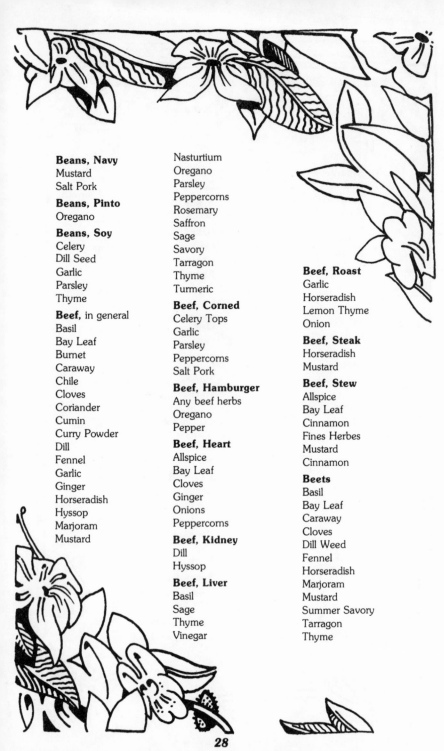

Beans, Navy
Mustard
Salt Pork

Beans, Pinto
Oregano

Beans, Soy
Celery
Dill Seed
Garlic
Parsley
Thyme

Beef, in general
Basil
Bay Leaf
Burnet
Caraway
Chile
Cloves
Coriander
Cumin
Curry Powder
Dill
Fennel
Garlic
Ginger
Horseradish
Hyssop
Marjoram
Mustard

Nasturtium
Oregano
Parsley
Peppercorns
Rosemary
Saffron
Sage
Savory
Tarragon
Thyme
Turmeric

Beef, Corned
Celery Tops
Garlic
Parsley
Peppercorns
Salt Pork

Beef, Hamburger
Any beef herbs
Oregano
Pepper

Beef, Heart
Allspice
Bay Leaf
Cloves
Ginger
Onions
Peppercorns

Beef, Kidney
Dill
Hyssop

Beef, Liver
Basil
Sage
Thyme
Vinegar

Beef, Roast
Garlic
Horseradish
Lemon Thyme
Onion

Beef, Steak
Horseradish
Mustard

Beef, Stew
Allspice
Bay Leaf
Cinnamon
Fines Herbes
Mustard
Cinnamon

Beets
Basil
Bay Leaf
Caraway
Cloves
Dill Weed
Fennel
Horseradish
Marjoram
Mustard
Summer Savory
Tarragon
Thyme

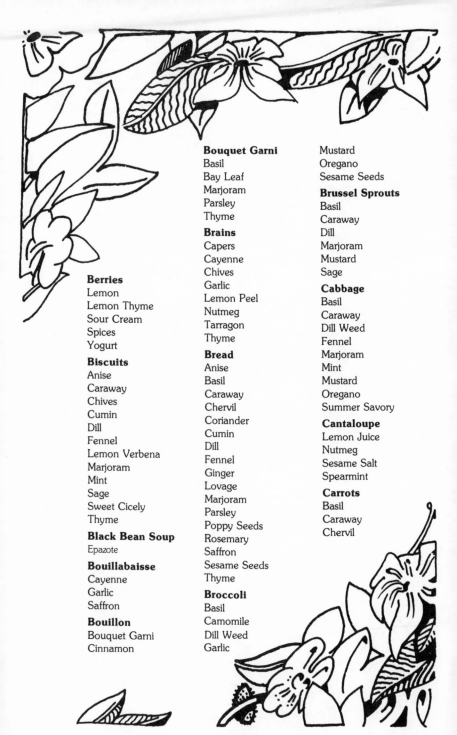

Berries
Lemon
Lemon Thyme
Sour Cream
Spices
Yogurt

Biscuits
Anise
Caraway
Chives
Cumin
Dill
Fennel
Lemon Verbena
Marjoram
Mint
Sage
Sweet Cicely
Thyme

Black Bean Soup
Epazote

Bouillabaisse
Cayenne
Garlic
Saffron

Bouillon
Bouquet Garni
Cinnamon

Bouquet Garni
Basil
Bay Leaf
Marjoram
Parsley
Thyme

Brains
Capers
Cayenne
Chives
Garlic
Lemon Peel
Nutmeg
Tarragon
Thyme

Bread
Anise
Basil
Caraway
Chervil
Coriander
Cumin
Dill
Fennel
Ginger
Lovage
Marjoram
Parsley
Poppy Seeds
Rosemary
Saffron
Sesame Seeds
Thyme

Broccoli
Basil
Camomile
Dill Weed
Garlic
Mustard
Oregano
Sesame Seeds

Brussel Sprouts
Basil
Caraway
Dill
Marjoram
Mustard
Sage

Cabbage
Basil
Caraway
Dill Weed
Fennel
Marjoram
Mint
Mustard
Oregano
Summer Savory

Cantaloupe
Lemon Juice
Nutmeg
Sesame Salt
Spearmint

Carrots
Basil
Caraway
Chervil

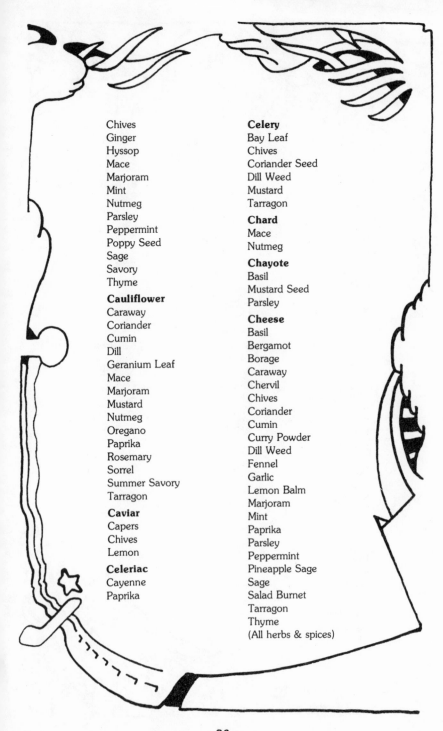

Chives
Ginger
Hyssop
Mace
Marjoram
Mint
Nutmeg
Parsley
Peppermint
Poppy Seed
Sage
Savory
Thyme

Cauliflower
Caraway
Coriander
Cumin
Dill
Geranium Leaf
Mace
Marjoram
Mustard
Nutmeg
Oregano
Paprika
Rosemary
Sorrel
Summer Savory
Tarragon

Caviar
Capers
Chives
Lemon

Celeriac
Cayenne
Paprika

Celery
Bay Leaf
Chives
Coriander Seed
Dill Weed
Mustard
Tarragon

Chard
Mace
Nutmeg

Chayote
Basil
Mustard Seed
Parsley

Cheese
Basil
Bergamot
Borage
Caraway
Chervil
Chives
Coriander
Cumin
Curry Powder
Dill Weed
Fennel
Garlic
Lemon Balm
Marjoram
Mint
Paprika
Parsley
Peppermint
Pineapple Sage
Sage
Salad Burnet
Tarragon
Thyme
(All herbs & spices)

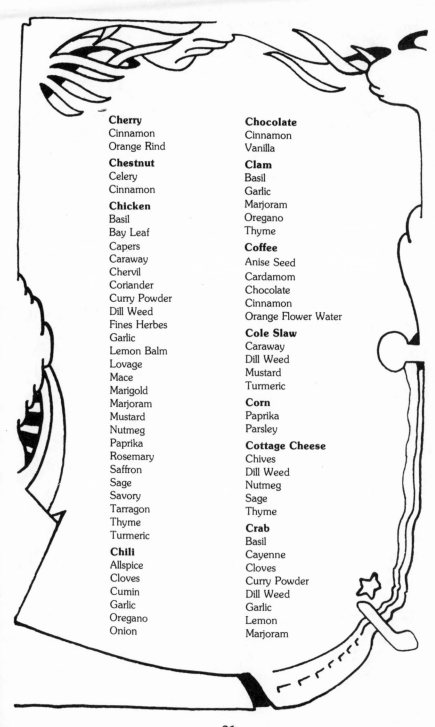

Cherry
Cinnamon
Orange Rind

Chestnut
Celery
Cinnamon

Chicken
Basil
Bay Leaf
Capers
Caraway
Chervil
Coriander
Curry Powder
Dill Weed
Fines Herbes
Garlic
Lemon Balm
Lovage
Mace
Marigold
Marjoram
Mustard
Nutmeg
Paprika
Rosemary
Saffron
Sage
Savory
Tarragon
Thyme
Turmeric

Chili
Allspice
Cloves
Cumin
Garlic
Oregano
Onion

Chocolate
Cinnamon
Vanilla

Clam
Basil
Garlic
Marjoram
Oregano
Thyme

Coffee
Anise Seed
Cardamom
Chocolate
Cinnamon
Orange Flower Water

Cole Slaw
Caraway
Dill Weed
Mustard
Turmeric

Corn
Paprika
Parsley

Cottage Cheese
Chives
Dill Weed
Nutmeg
Sage
Thyme

Crab
Basil
Cayenne
Cloves
Curry Powder
Dill Weed
Garlic
Lemon
Marjoram

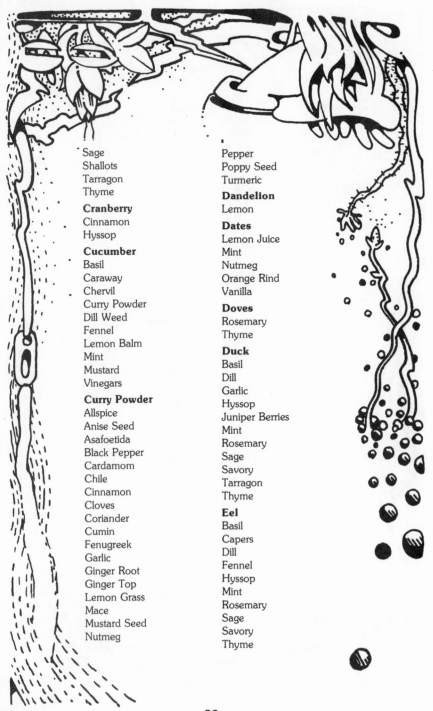

Sage
Shallots
Tarragon
Thyme

Cranberry
Cinnamon
Hyssop

Cucumber
Basil
Caraway
Chervil
Curry Powder
Dill Weed
Fennel
Lemon Balm
Mint
Mustard
Vinegars

Curry Powder
Allspice
Anise Seed
Asafoetida
Black Pepper
Cardamom
Chile
Cinnamon
Cloves
Coriander
Cumin
Fenugreek
Garlic
Ginger Root
Ginger Top
Lemon Grass
Mace
Mustard Seed
Nutmeg

Pepper
Poppy Seed
Turmeric

Dandelion
Lemon

Dates
Lemon Juice
Mint
Nutmeg
Orange Rind
Vanilla

Doves
Rosemary
Thyme

Duck
Basil
Dill
Garlic
Hyssop
Juniper Berries
Mint
Rosemary
Sage
Savory
Tarragon
Thyme

Eel
Basil
Capers
Dill
Fennel
Hyssop
Mint
Rosemary
Sage
Savory
Thyme

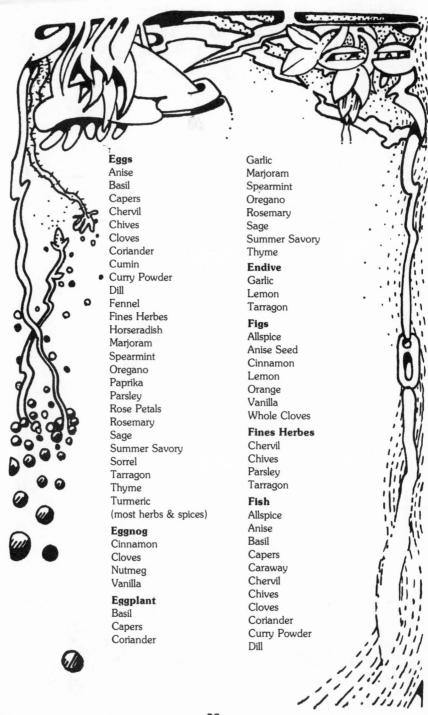

Eggs
Anise
Basil
Capers
Chervil
Chives
Cloves
Coriander
Cumin
Curry Powder
Dill
Fennel
Fines Herbes
Horseradish
Marjoram
Spearmint
Oregano
Paprika
Parsley
Rose Petals
Rosemary
Sage
Summer Savory
Sorrel
Tarragon
Thyme
Turmeric
(most herbs & spices)

Eggnog
Cinnamon
Cloves
Nutmeg
Vanilla

Eggplant
Basil
Capers
Coriander
Garlic
Marjoram
Spearmint
Oregano
Rosemary
Sage
Summer Savory
Thyme

Endive
Garlic
Lemon
Tarragon

Figs
Allspice
Anise Seed
Cinnamon
Lemon
Orange
Vanilla
Whole Cloves

Fines Herbes
Chervil
Chives
Parsley
Tarragon

Fish
Allspice
Anise
Basil
Capers
Caraway
Chervil
Chives
Cloves
Coriander
Curry Powder
Dill

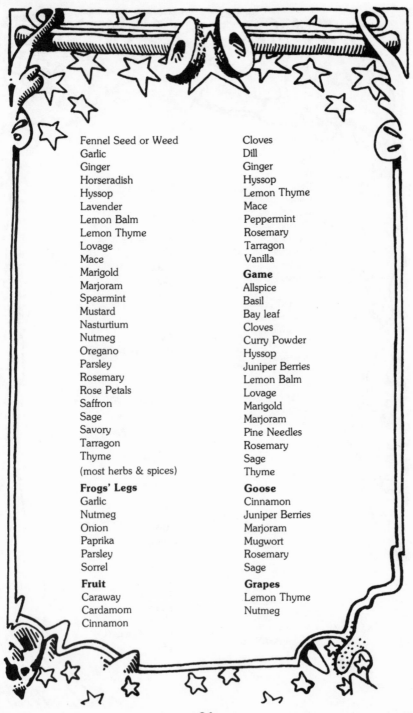

Fennel Seed or Weed
Garlic
Ginger
Horseradish
Hyssop
Lavender
Lemon Balm
Lemon Thyme
Lovage
Mace
Marigold
Marjoram
Spearmint
Mustard
Nasturtium
Nutmeg
Oregano
Parsley
Rosemary
Rose Petals
Saffron
Sage
Savory
Tarragon
Thyme
(most herbs & spices)

Frogs' Legs
Garlic
Nutmeg
Onion
Paprika
Parsley
Sorrel

Fruit
Caraway
Cardamom
Cinnamon

Cloves
Dill
Ginger
Hyssop
Lemon Thyme
Mace
Peppermint
Rosemary
Tarragon
Vanilla

Game
Allspice
Basil
Bay leaf
Cloves
Curry Powder
Hyssop
Juniper Berries
Lemon Balm
Lovage
Marigold
Marjoram
Pine Needles
Rosemary
Sage
Thyme

Goose
Cinnamon
Juniper Berries
Marjoram
Mugwort
Rosemary
Sage

Grapes
Lemon Thyme
Nutmeg

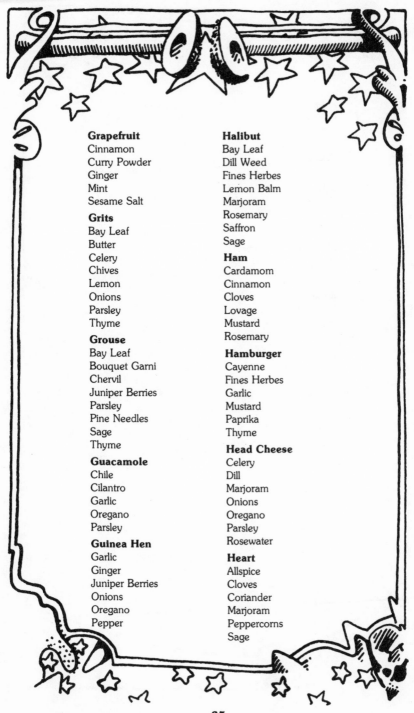

Grapefruit
Cinnamon
Curry Powder
Ginger
Mint
Sesame Salt

Grits
Bay Leaf
Butter
Celery
Chives
Lemon
Onions
Parsley
Thyme

Grouse
Bay Leaf
Bouquet Garni
Chervil
Juniper Berries
Parsley
Pine Needles
Sage
Thyme

Guacamole
Chile
Cilantro
Garlic
Oregano
Parsley

Guinea Hen
Garlic
Ginger
Juniper Berries
Onions
Oregano
Pepper

Halibut
Bay Leaf
Dill Weed
Fines Herbes
Lemon Balm
Marjoram
Rosemary
Saffron
Sage

Ham
Cardamom
Cinnamon
Cloves
Lovage
Mustard
Rosemary

Hamburger
Cayenne
Fines Herbes
Garlic
Mustard
Paprika
Thyme

Head Cheese
Celery
Dill
Marjoram
Onions
Oregano
Parsley
Rosewater

Heart
Allspice
Cloves
Coriander
Marjoram
Peppercorns
Sage

Herring
Dill Weed
Lemon Thyme
Onions
Sour Cream
Vinegar

Jam
Borage
Elderberries
Ginger
Juniper Berries
Lemon Balm
Roses
Violets

Jelly
Borage
Elderberries
Flowers
Geranium Leaves
Ginger
Lemon Balm
Mace
Rosemary
Rose Petals
Violets

Jerusalem Artichokes
Bay Leaves

Kidneys
Caraway
Dill
Fines Herbes
Hyssop

Kohlrabi
Fines Herbes

Lamb
Allspice
Basil

Bay Leaf
Capers
Caraway
Cinnamon
Cloves
Coriander Seed or Leaf
Cumin
Curry Powder
Dill Weed
Fennel Seed
Garlic
Ginger
Hyssop
Lemon Balm
Mace
Marigold
Marjoram
Nasturtiums
Oregano
Peppermint
Rosemary
Spearmint
Tarragon
Thyme
Turmeric

Leeks
Basil
Chervil
Sage
Tarragon

Lentils
Bay Leaf
Dillweed
Fennel
Garlic
Spearmint
Oregano
Savory
Tarragon

Liver
Basil
Coriander
Cumin
Fines Herbes
Marjoram
Sage
Savory
Thyme

Lobster
Cayenne
Garlic
Lemon
Lemon Thyme
Onion
Oregano
Tarragon
Turmeric

Macaroni
(see Pasta)

Mayonnaise
Cayenne
Garlic
Lemon
Lovage
Mustard
Parsley

Meat (See Also Beef)
Cloves
Fines Herbes
Garlic
Juniper Berries
Lemon Balm
Lovage
Nutmeg
Thyme
(all herbs & spices)

Melons
Brie Cheese
Orange
Peppermint
Sesame Salt
(spices)

Milk
Cinnamon
Dill Seed
Fennel Seed
Nutmeg
"Oak Leaf" Geranium

Mincemeat
Apples
Cinnamon
Cloves
Lemon Peel
Mace
Nutmeg
Orange Peel
Pepper, Black

Mushrooms
Fines Herbes
Hyssop
Lemon Balm
Marjoram
Spearmint
Primrose Petals
Tarragon
Thyme

Mussels
Basil
Capers
Celery
Chervil
Garlic
Oregano
Parsley

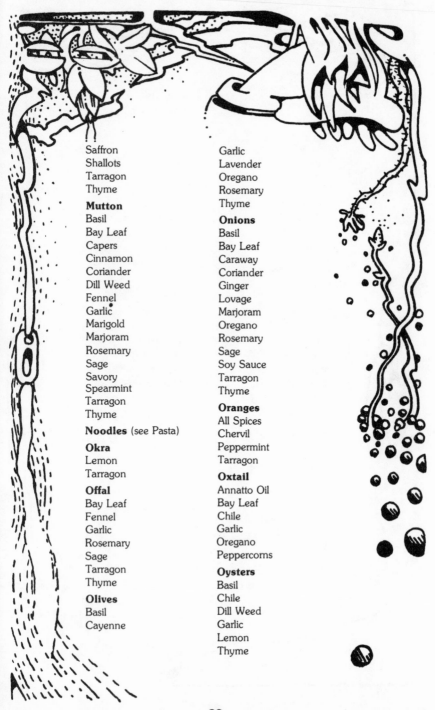

Saffron
Shallots
Tarragon
Thyme

Mutton
Basil
Bay Leaf
Capers
Cinnamon
Coriander
Dill Weed
Fennel
Garlic
Marigold
Marjoram
Rosemary
Sage
Savory
Spearmint
Tarragon
Thyme

Noodles (see Pasta)

Okra
Lemon
Tarragon

Offal
Bay Leaf
Fennel
Garlic
Rosemary
Sage
Tarragon
Thyme

Olives
Basil
Cayenne

Garlic
Lavender
Oregano
Rosemary
Thyme

Onions
Basil
Bay Leaf
Caraway
Coriander
Ginger
Lovage
Marjoram
Oregano
Rosemary
Sage
Soy Sauce
Tarragon
Thyme

Oranges
All Spices
Chervil
Peppermint
Tarragon

Oxtail
Annatto Oil
Bay Leaf
Chile
Garlic
Oregano
Peppercorns

Oysters
Basil
Chile
Dill Weed
Garlic
Lemon
Thyme

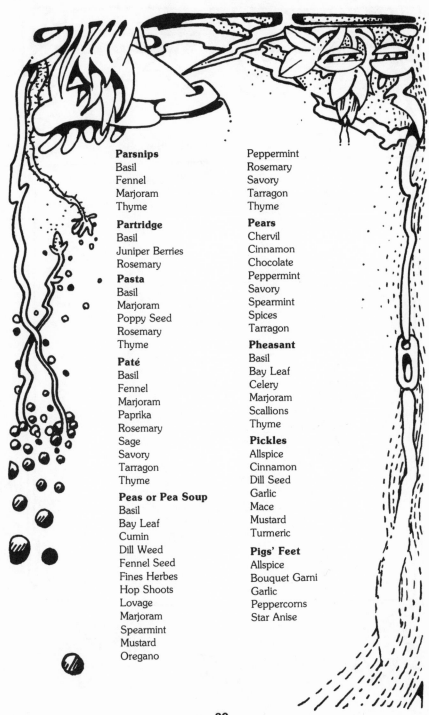

Parsnips
Basil
Fennel
Marjoram
Thyme

Partridge
Basil
Juniper Berries
Rosemary

Pasta
Basil
Marjoram
Poppy Seed
Rosemary
Thyme

Paté
Basil
Fennel
Marjoram
Paprika
Rosemary
Sage
Savory
Tarragon
Thyme

Peas or Pea Soup
Basil
Bay Leaf
Cumin
Dill Weed
Fennel Seed
Fines Herbes
Hop Shoots
Lovage
Marjoram
Spearmint
Mustard
Oregano

Peppermint
Rosemary
Savory
Tarragon
Thyme

Pears
Chervil
Cinnamon
Chocolate
Peppermint
Savory
Spearmint
Spices
Tarragon

Pheasant
Basil
Bay Leaf
Celery
Marjoram
Scallions
Thyme

Pickles
Allspice
Cinnamon
Dill Seed
Garlic
Mace
Mustard
Turmeric

Pigs' Feet
Allspice
Bouquet Garni
Garlic
Peppercorns
Star Anise

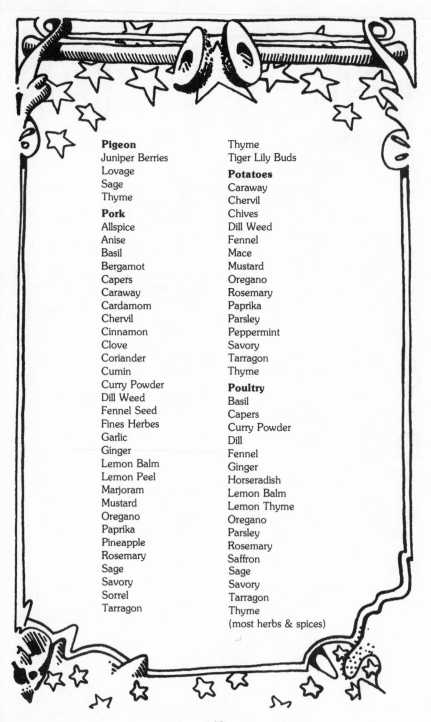

Pigeon
Juniper Berries
Lovage
Sage
Thyme

Pork
Allspice
Anise
Basil
Bergamot
Capers
Caraway
Cardamom
Chervil
Cinnamon
Clove
Coriander
Cumin
Curry Powder
Dill Weed
Fennel Seed
Fines Herbes
Garlic
Ginger
Lemon Balm
Lemon Peel
Marjoram
Mustard
Oregano
Paprika
Pineapple
Rosemary
Sage
Savory
Sorrel
Tarragon

Thyme
Tiger Lily Buds

Potatoes
Caraway
Chervil
Chives
Dill Weed
Fennel
Mace
Mustard
Oregano
Rosemary
Paprika
Parsley
Peppermint
Savory
Tarragon
Thyme

Poultry
Basil
Capers
Curry Powder
Dill
Fennel
Ginger
Horseradish
Lemon Balm
Lemon Thyme
Oregano
Parsley
Rosemary
Saffron
Sage
Savory
Tarragon
Thyme
(most herbs & spices)

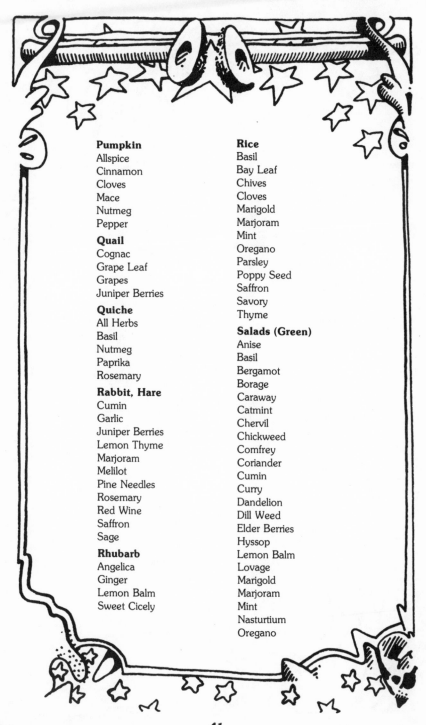

Pumpkin
Allspice
Cinnamon
Cloves
Mace
Nutmeg
Pepper

Quail
Cognac
Grape Leaf
Grapes
Juniper Berries

Quiche
All Herbs
Basil
Nutmeg
Paprika
Rosemary

Rabbit, Hare
Cumin
Garlic
Juniper Berries
Lemon Thyme
Marjoram
Melilot
Pine Needles
Rosemary
Red Wine
Saffron
Sage

Rhubarb
Angelica
Ginger
Lemon Balm
Sweet Cicely

Rice
Basil
Bay Leaf
Chives
Cloves
Marigold
Marjoram
Mint
Oregano
Parsley
Poppy Seed
Saffron
Savory
Thyme

Salads (Green)
Anise
Basil
Bergamot
Borage
Caraway
Catmint
Chervil
Chickweed
Comfrey
Coriander
Cumin
Curry
Dandelion
Dill Weed
Elder Berries
Hyssop
Lemon Balm
Lovage
Marigold
Marjoram
Mint
Nasturtium
Oregano

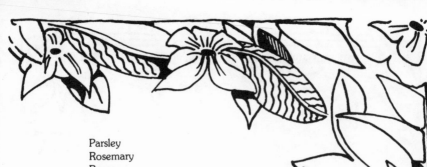

Parsley
Rosemary
Roses
Savory
Sweet Cicely
Tarragon
Violets
(all herbs & spices)
(See individual vegetables)

Salad (Fruit)
(all spices)
Lemon Thyme

Salmon
Bay Leaf
Dill Weed
Fennel
Marjoram
Rosemary
Sage
Savory
Turmeric

Salsify
Celery
Marjoram
Tarragon

Sardines
Garlic
Lemon
Mustard
Vinegar

Sausage
Basil
Marjoram
Oregano
Sage

Sauerkraut
Caraway
Dill Seed
Fennel
Juniper Berries

Scallops
Lavender Cotton
Tarragon
Thyme

Seafood & Shellfish
Basil
Dill Weed
Fennel
Lemon Balm
Mustard
Nutmeg
Oregano
Parsley
Rosemary
Saffron
Savory
Tarragon
Thyme
Turmeric

Shrimp
Basil
Bay Leaf
Chile
Coriander
Dill Weed

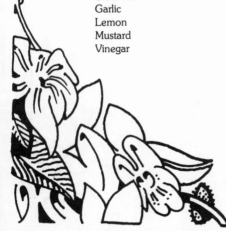

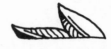

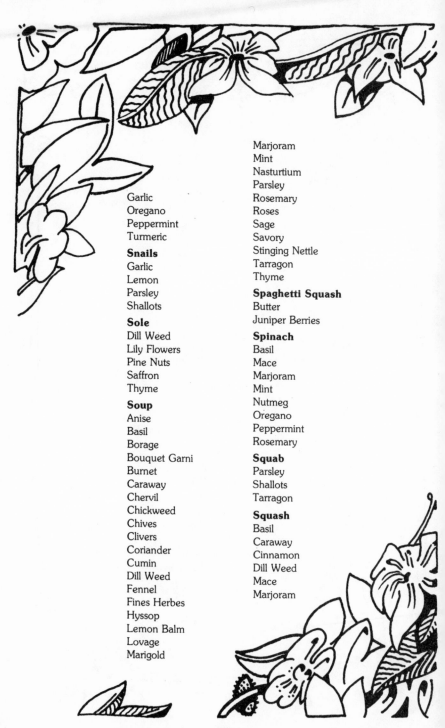

Garlic
Oregano
Peppermint
Turmeric

Snails
Garlic
Lemon
Parsley
Shallots

Sole
Dill Weed
Lily Flowers
Pine Nuts
Saffron
Thyme

Soup
Anise
Basil
Borage
Bouquet Garni
Burnet
Caraway
Chervil
Chickweed
Chives
Clivers
Coriander
Cumin
Dill Weed
Fennel
Fines Herbes
Hyssop
Lemon Balm
Lovage
Marigold

Marjoram
Mint
Nasturtium
Parsley
Rosemary
Roses
Sage
Savory
Stinging Nettle
Tarragon
Thyme

Spaghetti Squash
Butter
Juniper Berries

Spinach
Basil
Mace
Marjoram
Mint
Nutmeg
Oregano
Peppermint
Rosemary

Squab
Parsley
Shallots
Tarragon

Squash
Basil
Caraway
Cinnamon
Dill Weed
Mace
Marjoram

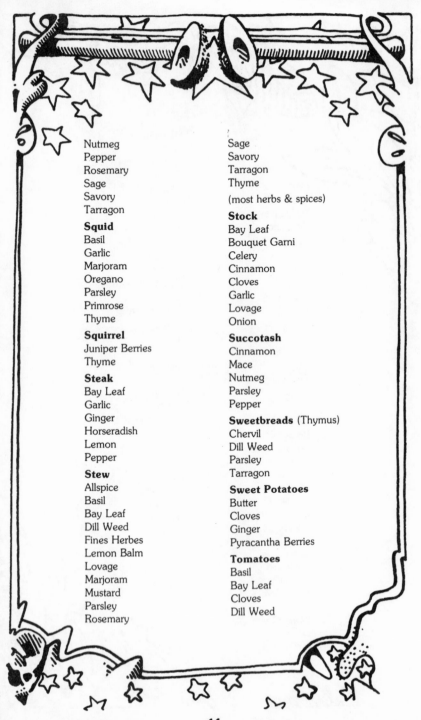

Nutmeg
Pepper
Rosemary
Sage
Savory
Tarragon

Squid
Basil
Garlic
Marjoram
Oregano
Parsley
Primrose
Thyme

Squirrel
Juniper Berries
Thyme

Steak
Bay Leaf
Garlic
Ginger
Horseradish
Lemon
Pepper

Stew
Allspice
Basil
Bay Leaf
Dill Weed
Fines Herbes
Lemon Balm
Lovage
Marjoram
Mustard
Parsley
Rosemary

Sage
Savory
Tarragon
Thyme
(most herbs & spices)

Stock
Bay Leaf
Bouquet Garni
Celery
Cinnamon
Cloves
Garlic
Lovage
Onion

Succotash
Cinnamon
Mace
Nutmeg
Parsley
Pepper

Sweetbreads (Thymus)
Chervil
Dill Weed
Parsley
Tarragon

Sweet Potatoes
Butter
Cloves
Ginger
Pyracantha Berries

Tomatoes
Basil
Bay Leaf
Cloves
Dill Weed

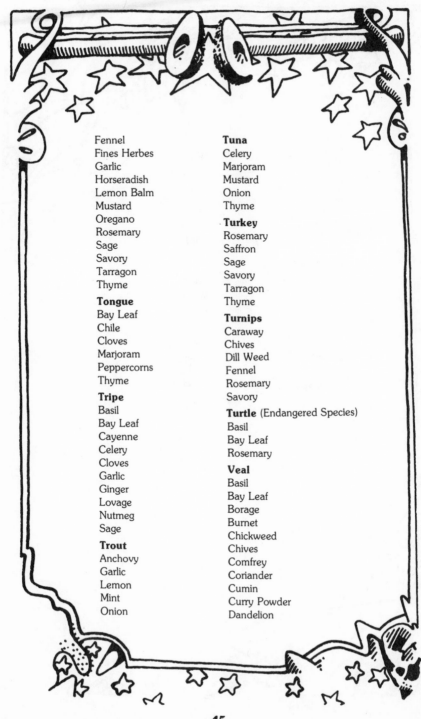

Fennel
Fines Herbes
Garlic
Horseradish
Lemon Balm
Mustard
Oregano
Rosemary
Sage
Savory
Tarragon
Thyme

Tongue
Bay Leaf
Chile
Cloves
Marjoram
Peppercorns
Thyme

Tripe
Basil
Bay Leaf
Cayenne
Celery
Cloves
Garlic
Ginger
Lovage
Nutmeg
Sage

Trout
Anchovy
Garlic
Lemon
Mint
Onion

Tuna
Celery
Marjoram
Mustard
Onion
Thyme

Turkey
Rosemary
Saffron
Sage
Savory
Tarragon
Thyme

Turnips
Caraway
Chives
Dill Weed
Fennel
Rosemary
Savory

Turtle (Endangered Species)
Basil
Bay Leaf
Rosemary

Veal
Basil
Bay Leaf
Borage
Burnet
Chickweed
Chives
Comfrey
Coriander
Cumin
Curry Powder
Dandelion

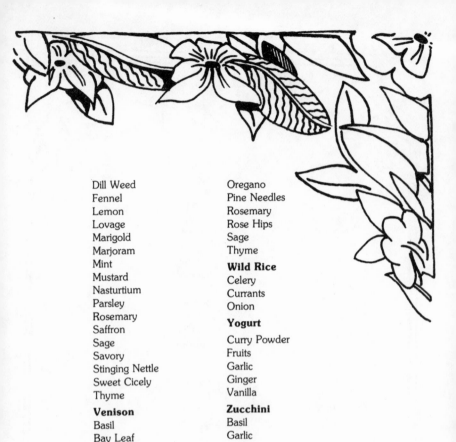

Dill Weed
Fennel
Lemon
Lovage
Marigold
Marjoram
Mint
Mustard
Nasturtium
Parsley
Rosemary
Saffron
Sage
Savory
Stinging Nettle
Sweet Cicely
Thyme

Venison
Basil
Bay Leaf
Juniper Berries
Marjoram

Oregano
Pine Needles
Rosemary
Rose Hips
Sage
Thyme

Wild Rice
Celery
Currants
Onion

Yogurt
Curry Powder
Fruits
Garlic
Ginger
Vanilla

Zucchini
Basil
Garlic
Marjoram
Peppermint

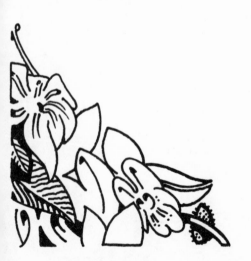

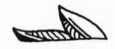

A Culinary Glossary of Terms

Absorbent. A substance that can absorb another, such as a piece of bread wiped across cool soup to suck up the grease that rises to the top, or a sponge used to soak up liquid.

Al Dente. An Italian word meaning "to the tooth" and applied to the degree to which pasta is cooked, that is, not soft and sticky but so the teeth can still grab on and get a taste.

Alterative. A vague term in herbalism which means a substance that affects the blood and changes it slowly from an unhealthy or unbalanced state to one that is healthy and/or balanced.

Anodyne. A pain killer; sometimes herbal liqueurs act as pain killers when taken internally.

Antipyretic. A substance that reduces fever; eating chiles can sometimes do this as they make you sweat (act as diaphoretics) which helps adjust the body's thermal mechanism.

Antiseptic. A substance that inhibits the growth of microorganisms on living tissues.

Aromatherapy. Using the volatile oils of a plant to treat mental and physical ailments.

Aromatic. Something that smells good, or ingredients that give scent and flavor to a recipe.

Aromemories. Memories associated with various scents, and in this book particularly with the various cooking scents.

Astringent. A substance that stops an excess of liquid from exuding from a wound, or a product used in cosmetics that "closes" the pores.

Au Gratin. A food that has been moistened with liquid, stock, cream, covered with crumbs and butter or cheese, and then baked or broiled until the top is browned.

Au Jus. Meat that is served in its own cooking juices.

Au Lait. Food served with milk, such as coffee.

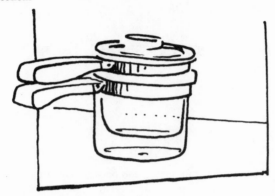

Bain-Marie. A type of water bath (double boiler) used for scrambling eggs and making fine sauces or fine cosmetics. The top pan fits deeply into the bottom pan which holds the boiling water. The boiling water is underneath, as well as around the sides of the top pan.

Bake. To cook by dry heat in the oven.

Baste. To spoon or brush melted fat or hot liquid over food as it roasts in the oven or is broiled. Basting should be done several times while the food cooks to keep it tender and juicy, and to keep it from burning.

Beat. To stir vigorously with a circular or figure-eight motion, usually using a wire whisk or an egg-beater. It gives lightness to the mixture.

Blend. To beat or stir a mixture of foods until they are combined and smooth.

Boil. When the liquid is bubbling and at the boiling point (212°F).

Bouquet Garni. A bunch of Thyme, Bay leaf, and Marjoram, tied round with a sprig of Parsley and tied in a muslin bag or with a string. The Bouquet Garni is used to give flavor to food and is removed before serving.

Bruise. To mash, crush, pulverize, or rub between your fingers a plant or leaf to extract its properties. A mortar and pestle can also be used.

Casserole. A mixture of different foods cooked in a heavy Dutch oven and placed in an oven to cook slowly over low heat.

Chill. To cool in the refrigerator or on ice. Do not freeze.

Chop. To cut into small to medium-size uneven pieces with a knife.

Clarify. To remove impurities by melting the substance that has fat in it with water, boiling it up so that the fat rises, and then removing the fat and straining the liquid/stock.

Condiment. A flavored sauce, a particular seasoning, a relish, or a spice.

Cool. To lower to room temperature.

Court Bouillon. A stock made from water, vegetables, wine, herbs, and parts of fish in which to poach fish and which, when strained, can be used in sauces.

Crudities. Raw, cut vegetables served as hors d'oeuvres.

Cuisine. Literally means the kitchen, but also cooking.

Decoction. A liquid extract of the hard parts of plants, obtained by boiling. One to four ounces of the plant is added to twenty ounces of water, brought to a boil and simmered 5–20 minutes. The liquid can be strained and can be used internally or externally as a medicine, cosmetic, in fomentations, poultices, or plasters.

Demulcent. A soothing substance taken internally.

Deodorant. A substance used to inhibit or get rid of nasty odors.

Diaphoretic. A substance that makes you sweat, and if it also makes you urinate more, it is called a diuretic.

Dissolve. To melt a solid substance by mixing it into a liquid substance. The word is used culinarily and medicinally.

Diuretic. A substance which when taken internally causes more and frequent urination.

Elixir. A sweetened alcoholic or non-alcoholic substance. It is often about 25% alcohol.

Emollient. A soothing substance used externally.

Emulsion. A substance made of totally disparate ingredients which, if combined properly, will stay combined. Mayonnaise is considered an emulsion.

Essence. The substance of something, or an essential oil dissolved in alcohol.

Essential Oil. The volatile oils contained in a plant or plant part.

Fines Herbes. Chervil, Chives, Parsley, and Tarragon chopped and mixed together and used in flavoring foods.

Fold. To mix a light substance (such as beaten egg whites) into a heavier substance (such as cream sauce) in such a manner that the lightness is not lost (soufflé).

Fomentation. Cloths soaked in hot herbal decoctions or infusions and wrung out and applied to sore, infected, or aching areas to reduce inflammation or ease pain.

Fondue. A hot melted cheese and wine food made for dipping goodies.

Garnish. To decorate prepared foods in an attractive manner with herbs, etc.

Grate. To scrape or finely cut hard foods into small, even pieces by the use of a grater.

Grease. To coat a dish or food with a thin, even layer of fat or butter.

Herb. In herbalism *any* plant used for aromatic, culinary, medicinal, or cosmetic purpose is an Herb. This naturally takes into account ANY plant, tree, shrub, weed, flower, fungus, etc. In cooking, the word when used in the ingredients of recipes usually means the top of the plant as opposed to its root, i.e., there is such a thing as Fennel herb, Fennel seed, and Fennel root.

Herbal. A book in which many different kinds of plants are described, named, and their uses discussed.

Herbalism. The oldest healing art in the world; the art of healing by the use of nonpoisonous herbs, administered externally or internally, usually using the whole plant without eliminating any part.

Herbalist. One who uses plants for healing purposes.

Herbs (as opposed to Spices). Herbs are fragrant plants used culinarily to scent or flavor foods. All spices are herbs but not all herbs are necessarily spices. Cinnamon leaves would be considered an herb while Cinnamon bark would be considered a spice. Herbs are generally the soft parts of plants, the leaves, stems, flowers, whereas the spice is usually the hard parts of a plant, such as the bark, berries, seeds, and flower buds. (See also Spices.)

Hollandaise. A sauce made of egg yolks, butter, Lemon juice, and Tarragon.

Hors d'Oeuvre. Appetizers, the first course of a meal, or a snack of small things.

Infuse. To steep in warm liquid.

Infusion. The resultant liquid when boiling water is poured onto an herb. An infusion is usually made with the soft parts of a plant; one ounce of plant with twenty ounces of boiling water poured over, covered and let to steep five to twenty minutes. (See also Decoction.)

Julienne. When meat or vegetables are cut into matchstick-size pieces, usually ⅛-inch thick by 1½-inches long. A julienne is also a clear soup made with finely shredded vegetables floating in it.

Liqueur. A sweetened alcoholic beverage (like Cassis or Benedictine), or a solution of medicinal substances in water, as distinguished from a tincture.

Macerate. To soak or steep substances in liquid to soften, separate, or extract certain characteristics from them.

Marinate. To soak raw foods in an herbed and spiced liquid or oil (marinade) to flavor and/or tenderize them.

Medicinal. A substance used in treating physical or mental disease.

Mellite. An infusion or decoction mixed or made with enough honey to preserve it.

Minestrone. A thick vegetable-laden Italian soup.

Nervine. A substance to soothe the nerves.

Pasta. Spaghetti, macaroni, or noodles.

Pâté. Ground, pounded, seasoned meat or fish.

Phytotherapy. The use of plants in healing.

Poach. To cook gently in quivering but not boiling liquid.

Poultice. A substance applied directly to the flesh and covered by a hot cloth that has usually been soaked in a hot herbal liquid; used to ease pain, cause increased circulation, or to heal wounds.

Pound. To reduce a substance to a paste using a mortar and pestle.

Purée. Meat, vegetables, or fruits treated in such a way, by cooking, straining, or blending, that they resemble a thick cream (like tomato paste).

Quiche. A cheese, egg, or cream custard baked in a pie shell and seasoned.

Ramekin. A small, individual-size baking dish, suitable for baked or shirred eggs or casseroles.

Render. To melt fat to clarify it, usually done slowly in the oven, the cut-up fat pieces then boiled in water and strained, cooled and separated when solidified.

Roast. Cooking with direct heat.

Sauté. To gently but quickly brown or tenderize food in a very small quantity of hot fat (oil or butter) in a skillet or sauce pan.

Sedative. A calming or soothing substance.

Sieve. A kitchen container with holes of one size or another through which food is forced in order to obtain a purée. Also used to separate solids from liquids.

Simmer. To cook gently so that the substance is always below the boiling point, with just a bubble or two coming to the surface. Simmering food quivers when it cooks.

Soufflé. An egg dish, cooked in the oven, which rises lightly above its straight-sided cooking dish. When pierced it belches air with a distinct pouf.

Spices. These are the dried parts of very aromatic plants that usually make their home in the tropics. Spices are usually hard parts of plants such as pieces of bark (Cinnamon), roots (Ginger), flower buds (Cloves), or berries (Pepper). (See also Herbs.)

Steam. In cooking, steaming food causes it to cook slowly without loss of nutrients and is usually done by placing a trivet or sieve in the bottom of a pot to hold the food above the heat and boiling water that creates the steam. The pot is kept covered to contain the steam. In beauty care, steaming is done to face or body to cause sweating which increases circulation. This helps to open the pores and relieve them of their accumulation of dirt and toxins. Steaming the skin hydrates by adding moisture.

Stock. The liquid that results from simmering a variety of foods and seasonings together in a quantity of water, and then straining. The foods are used to flavor the liquid and are usually discarded, while the stock goes on to make heavenly soups. Stocks are often made of used-up bones.

Syrup. An infusion or decoction made with sugar to sweeten and preserve it, also the boiled down product of tree sap, such as Maple syrup.

Tea. A simple beverage of herb and boiling water (1 t. to 1 C.) that is infused only for a few minutes to extract only the volatile essence of the plant. A tea can be made into a medicinal brew by using more herb to the water and infusing for a longer period of time. Tea is also the product that results from drying and fermenting leaves of *Thea sinensis* (also called India Tea).

Tenderize. The breaking down of the tough fibers of meat (or abalone) by beating, heating, macerating, rolling, or marinating.

Tisane. A tea made of flowers or fragrant herbs.

Vinaigrette. A dressing or sauce made of oil, vinegar, Mustard, a bit of sugar, and chopped herbs and spices, usually to season meat, salad, or cooked vegetables.

Water Bath. Also known as a *bain-marie*. A container of water in which another pan is placed containing the substance being cooked; used for cooking delicate or sensitive ingredients which require low heat.

Whisk. Beating with a wire or balloon whisk in a quick and circular motion. Used to incorporate air into the ingredients and imperative for making soufflés, or to give egg whites their lightest, airiest, and smallest size air bubbles and greatest volume. It is best to use a copper bowl and a balloon whisk.

For further definitions of herbal terms, see *Herbs & Things: Jeanne Rose's Herbal* or *The Herbal Body Book* for body care preparation definitions. A few of the above definitions came from these books.

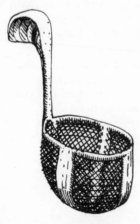

Chapter 3

The Organic Culinary Materia Medica
A description of the plants useful in the kitchen

Honor the healer for his services,
for the Lord created him.
His skill comes from the Most High,
and he is rewarded by kings.
The healer's knowledge gives him high standing
and wins him the admiration of the great.
THE LORD HAS CREATED MEDICINES FROM THE EARTH,
and a sensible man will not disparage them."

Apocrypha, Ecclesiasticus, Chapter 38

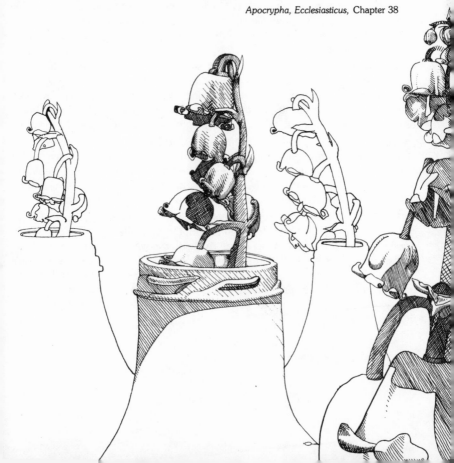

The substances marked ▲ have been known to have caused irritation, allergic reactions, or sensitivities in some people. However, all substances have been implicated to some degree in unpleasant reactions on someone, so it would behoove you to try just a little bit of a new plant externally, * (if you are prone to allergies) before you take it internally.

▲**Acacia, Gum** *(Acacia senegal)*, formed by an exudation of the cell wall, is slowly soluble in water. As with the leaves of some species, gum Acacia shows an acid reaction, is demulcent in action, and can be mixed with other ingredients to form a soothing food for inflammatory conditions of the digestive tract. Try mixing gum Acacia mucilage with Lemon juice and Apple pectin (Lemon-flavored Acacia gelatin) for diarrhea or stomach distress. I have also thought about the use of this acid-type gum mixed with Vitamin C and Comfrey root extract as a natural-type gel contraceptive. However, I have not as yet tried it although the possibility is infinitely interesting. M. Grieve in her book, *A Modern Herbal* (see Bibliography), says that gum Acacia, being highly nutritious, can be used as an exclusive drink in times of need, and that six ounces of the gum (or mucilage) can support an adult for twenty-four hours.

▲**Acacia,** flowers and leaves *(Acacia spp.)* are sometimes used in cookery where they have an acid reaction. Acacia flower fritters can be made using a batter of light beer and beaten egg whites. Some suggest dipping the flower sprays first in powdered sugar and cherry liqueur, letting them dry somewhat before dipping in the batter and frying. The fritters are then cooled and sprinkled with more powdered sugar.

▲**Agrimony** *(Agrimonia eupatoria)* is commonly called Stickwort because its seed vesicles have hooked hairs that stick onto clothes. It is used as a beverage tea to give tone to the bodily systems and to promote good assimilation of food. The flower spikes have an odor not unlike fresh Apricots, and these have been used to flavor beer or wine. It is often used by the French as a tisane to "purify" the blood.

▲**Alfalfa** *(Medicago sativa)* tea, especially when mixed with other herbs such as Dandelion and Parsley, is good to detoxify the body or during a fast. We normally do not eat Alfalfa herb, but who can eat an Avocado sandwich without delicious fresh Alfalfa sprouts? These and other sprouts should definitely be added to everyone's diet as they are an excellent source of vitamins and minerals. For raw food addicts, Alfalfa and Mung Bean sprouts are extremely important in the diet as an abundant source of protein. Skinny people should drink a daily dose of Alfalfa herb infusion to provide nutrients.

*See Jeanne Rose, The *Herbal Body Book,* p. 41.

Alexander *(Smyrnium Olusatrum)* is also known as Black Lovage. The buds are used in salad vinegars and in salads. Culpeper says "It is an herb of Jupiter, and therefore friendly to nature, for it warmeth a cold ftomach, and openeth ftoppings of the liver, and wonderfully helpeth the fpleen. . . . If boiled in wine, or bruifed and taken in wine, it is alfo effectual againft the biting of ferpents. And now you know what Alexander pottage* is good for, that you may no longer eat it out of ignorance, but out of knowledge." The buds can be boiled as a vegetable or used to flavor soups.

*A mess of vegetables, cooked and seasoned.

▲**Allspice** *(Pimenta officinalis)* is also called Pimento. It is a spice of which the fruit and particularly the shell, when dried, are used in cookery. This spice tastes rather like a combination of Pepper, Cinnamon, Cloves, and Juniper berries with a bit of Nutmeg thrown in. It is used as an aromatic stimulant to the digestive tract; a delicious drink can be made for this purpose by pouring 1 pint of boiling water over a small handful of crushed Allspice berries and infusing for 10–20 minutes. Add Lemon juice and a few Cloves, stir with a stick of Cinnamon, add rum if you like and drink. And, of course, you are probably familiar with the use of Allspice in Curry powder, pastries and Apple butter.

Almond *(Prunus dulcis)* is so familiar to all of us that it almost seems unnecessary to mention it. Almond meal makes an excellent facial mask to tone and clarify the complexion. Some authorities mention the use of Almond meal as a food for diabetics. Almonds can be eaten whole or added to any number of culinary dishes.

When I was a child we always had almond trees surrounding our house, and my childhood was truly enhanced through the knowledge of these trees. How else could I have become familiar with the tent caterpillar and its habits, or the clear squishy green color of its insides. The smell of Almond blossoms is still clear to me, and the memory of the strong bitter taste of Almond honey can still curl my lips.

California grows a very large percentage of the world's Almonds. In Palestine the appearance of Almond flowers in late winter heralds the awakening of Creation. Almonds can supply a very important part of a vegetarian's need for protein. Almond oil is an important oil for the complexion, is used in cooking certain dishes, and it will certainly enhance any salad.

There is a lovely legend of the creation of the Almond tree. The princess Phyllis and the prince Demophoon fell in love and decided to marry. First Demophoon had to put his affairs in order and so off he went, setting sail for home where he met another maid more fair (or so he thought) than his beloved Phyllis. Meanwhile Phyllis pined away in grief and died. But the Gods, admiring her constancy, changed her into an Almond tree. Demophoon, regretting his abandonment of Phyllis, returned to her, and, when the leafless, flowerless, and lonely tree was pointed out to him, he fell at its feet and embraced its trunk, his tears watering the roots, whereupon it burst into fragrant luxuriant bloom. Thus, in the language of flowers, it signifies constancy and hope.

When Almonds are pounded in water, the thin, pleasant tasting milky juice is collected and can be given to those who are sick as a substitute for cow's milk—this juice can be thickened by the addition of gum Acacia (gum Arabic). Barley water and mashed Almonds have been used as a food for those folks who suffer "stones" whether they are in the kidney, bladder or gall bladder. Culpeper mentions beating Almonds with sugar, Rosewater and Violets, and using this butter spread on toast as a good food for students to comfort and fortify their brains, give joy to the heart and cool a hot liver. And don't forget the flavoring ability of oil of Bitter Almonds. It is used in macaroons and the smell will surely remind you of Christmas and those delicious Italian cookies that are so prevalent then.

Aloe *(Aloe vera)* gel doesn't make a very tasty food but it certainly is useful to allay heat on or in the body. This means that it is a useful addition to the daily diet if you have ulcers or digestive disturbances (where there is a hot pain), or externally for sunburn. And who would have a kitchen where a live Aloe plant was not prominently displayed for its fantastic and immediate use on possible kitchen burns.

▲**Amaranth** *(Amaranthus spp.)*, has not much use yet economically, but some studies have been done concerning its economic value. It is easily digested, easily grown, tasty, full of protein, vitamins and minerals. It is exceedingly wholesome and easy to use; when cooked it tastes somewhat like Spinach and as such, is eaten as a vegetable. It is beneficial as a food for convalescents and as a cure for menstrual disorders. In ancient Greece it was used as a symbol of immortality to decorate tombs. (See *Prevention* Magazine, April 1976, p. 23, for a long article concerning the efficacy of Amaranth.)

Ambergris *(Physeter catadon)* is an exudate from this species of whale and is primarily used as a fixative in fine perfumes. However, in days past Ambergris was an ingredient in many culinary delicacies, especially those considered to be aphrodisiacal in nature.

Ambrette seed *(Hibiscus abelmoschus,* or *H. Moscheutes)* is also called Musk seed. It has a strong, penetrating odor very much like musk, is used in perfumery as a fixative, and in soups and pickles, or to give an unusual, delicious flavour to a coffee such as Yemen Mocha. The seeds can also be chewed as a breath freshener.

▲**Anemone** *(Anemone spp.)* flowers have often been used to dye Easter eggs.

Angelica *(Angelica Archangelica, A. sinensis)* has a use in all types of medicinal, cosmetic and culinary preparations. The roots should be dug up in autumn and can be candied, used to flavor liqueurs, boiled and eaten, or boiled with honey to make a pleasant cough syrup. The roots of the Chinese species, called *Dong quai,* are sliced transversely and eaten as a sweet, although they are more often given to nourish the female reproductive system and regulate the menstrual cycle. The essential oil of the roots is used in perfumery, medicine and in flavorings. Angelica stems can be used fresh in salads (especially good for flatulent personalities), in marmalades, or as a flavouring in drinks and wines. They can be candied and used in fruitcakes or confections. Angelica leaves are a good addition to fish, stewed rhubarb, salads, as a tea, and in potpourris. Angelica seeds are used in confectionery, as a flavouring agent in liqueurs, and in some herbal formulas.

▲**Angostura** *(Cusparia febrifuga)* bark has been known and used in South America and the West Indies to reduce fever, as its Latin name indicates. Commercially, we use it in aromatic bitters of the same name. Bitters are tinctures or extracts of bitter tasting aromatic herbs which combine the properties of an appetizer and a tonic. Putting a drop or two of a bitter such as Angostura on a cube of sugar and sucking it is an ancient but effective method of relieving stomach distress.

Anise *(Pimpinella Anisum;* Star Anise. *Illicium verum* or *I, anisatum)* seeds are much used in cooking as a quick glance in any cookbook will confirm. They are aromatic and of a group I call the "licorice" herbs because of their licorice-like scent. In former days, Anise seeds were used as payment for taxes, in spiced cakes to prevent indigestion, as flavoring for soups, in breads, liqueurs (Anisette), and to avert the Evil Eye. Anise leaves can be used to flavor vegetables, soups, green salads, fruit salads and pies, even wrapped around fish. Anise and Fennel seed tea is especially good for children suffering from diarrhea and for persons who have insomnia because of digestive disturbances. Star Anise belongs to the same order as the Magnolia tree, and thus we see it is an entirely different type of plant than the Umbelliferous Anise seed, but it is used in much the same way. It occurs more often in Oriental food, especially with Szechuan pepper. These seeds can be chewed to refresh the breath and soothe digestion, and they can be pounded and used in incense powders.

▲**Annatto** *(Bixa orellana)* has been used as a coloring agent in cosmetics and foods.

Apple *(Pyrus malus).* Skinner's book of *Myths and Legends* (see Bibliography) states that, "In the Norse legend Iduna kept a store of apples which the gods ate, thereby keeping themselves young." This points up one of the most important medicinal applications of this most delicious of fruits.

"To eat an apple 'pon going to bed
Will make the doctor beg his bread."

Eating raw apples will keep your teeth scrubbed clean, your complexion bright, your health vibrant, prolong your life and improve your spirit. So, forget about recipes using cooked apples; it's the fresh raw ones that will do all these wondrous things.

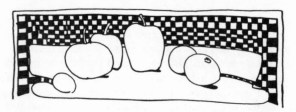

Apricot *(Prunus Armeniaca)* kernels furnish the product laetrile, called B-17, which is used in the treatment of cancer. I grew up on an Apricot orchard in Oakley, California. There my father told me it was very important to eat an occasional Apricot kernel, even though they were very bitter. We ate them to improve health. Apricots are delicious fruits that remind me of the sun. In every country and culture there are myths and legends surrounding the Apricot. Apricot oil is almost indistinguishable from Almond oil; it is used in cosmetics to soften the complexion, and also to improve the taste of many vegetable salads.

Arrach *(Atriplex hortensis* and *A. hastata)* is called Garden Arroche or Mountain Spinach, and is a member of the Goosefoot family. The leaves are "frequntly boil'd and eaten, like Coleworts, with salt Meats and in Sallads, and are cooling and moistening, rendring the Body soluble," (Miller, *Botanicum Officinale*). They probably contain a large amount of digestible iron, as does Good-King-Henry, another member of this Goosefoot family.

Arrowhead *(Sagittaria latifolia)* or Wapatoo is a water plant with an arrowhead-shaped leaf; the rhizome has been used as a food both in the raw state and cooked. It is also a medicinal plant for indigestion.

▲**Arrowroot** *(Maranta arundinacea)* was listed in the U.S.P. *(United States Pharmacopeia)* from 1820–1960. The starch from its rhizome is 87% carbohydrate, very easily digested, and is therefore a very good food for sick people or children. It was grown as food by several American Indian tribes and was once used as an antidote to wounds caused by arrow poison (hence the name). This starch should be mixed with a little cold water to a very smooth paste before any other liquid is added.

Artichoke *(Cynara Scolymus)* leaves are usually used medicinally, while the delicious immature flower head is eaten as a vegetable. There are many recipes for Artichokes——the best are the simplest (see Chapter 10. pg. 156). There is another food called the Jerusalem Artichoke *(Helianthus tuberosus)* which is the edible tuber of a type of sunflower. It is best sliced and eaten raw, in salads, or with a sauce of oil, Lemon, Garlic and Italian herbs (such as Marjoram). It is composed of a starch called inulin that is very good for diabetics.

Asafetida *(Ferula foetida)* has such a high stink like that of very old fermented garlic that it has been called Devil's Dung and also Food for the Gods. It is often used, with extreme discretion, as a component of Curry powder.

Asclepias (milkweeds) are notable as a food for the lovely monarch butterfly. Fresh flowers as well as the young shoots of some species are eaten by people.

Asparagus *(Asparagus officinalis)* spears are used in cosmetic preparations and medicinally as a laxative. One anti-aging book suggests that the frequent ingestion of Beets, Asparagus, Mushrooms, sardines and Onions will reduce the lines in your face, remove the circles under the eyes and, in general, make you feel better. It is the amino acid content of these foods that is important. One out of every seven persons has an enzyme variation that causes a potent pungent odor to the urine after they have eaten Asparagus. My entire family has this enzyme variation, and I have always wondered if we share any other genetic aberration with the rest of the world's potent Asparagus urine producers.

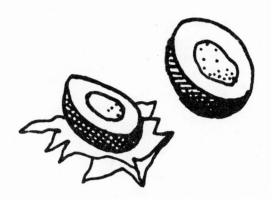

Avocado *(Persea americana)*. "The Alligator Pear contains Vitamins A, D, E, and potassium, sulfur, and chlorine." (Jeanne Rose, *The Herbal Body Book,* p. 51.) There are two main types of Avocado; the thin-skinned type available during the winter months that is rather tasteless because of its low oil content, and the thick-skinned type available during the summer months that is delicious and tasty because of its high oil content. We prefer the latter and use it exclusively in all salads, tortillas and guacamole. To ripen, put Avocadoes into a brown paper bag with a very ripe Apple. The Apple emits ripening gases retained in the paper bag which assist in the even ripening of the Avocadoes. You can ripen any fruit with this method, from Avocadoes to Pears, to Peaches to Melons.

Balm *(Melissa officinalis),* called Lemon Balm, Sweet Balm or Melissa is an excellent plant to grow because of its myriad uses. It has many applications in body care products (see *Herbal Body Book*), medicinal products (see Jeanne Rose, *Herbs & Things*), and in cooking. We like to add the leaves to any type of tea for a Lemony flavor, to herb butters, stuffings, sauces and desserts. Leg of lamb wrapped in Balm is delicious as is Rice with raisins and Balm served with a baked Garlic chicken. There is one cookbook that lists 12 recipes using Balm but the quantities are far too small for a really good taste. Try mixing twelve 4-inch long sprigs of fresh Balm that have been finely chopped, or put through a Parsley chopper, with 1 cup of yogurt in a bowl, cover and infuse, refrigerate for a few hours before eating. This Balm-flavored yogurt can be eaten as-is, used on fruit or mixed with Lemon juice as a dip for vegetables such as Artichokes. See Chapter 12. pg. 183 for a delightful Balm-wrapped fish recipe. Steep Balm in a white wine for several hours and use it as Gerarde states in *The Herball,* "Bawme drunke in wine is good against the bitings of venomous beasts, comforts the heart, and driveth away all melancholy and sad-nesse." The famous Carmelite water (available from Caswell-Massey in New York) is made from Balm, Angelica root, Lemon peel, Nutmeg and Clove; it has been used for headache and nervous afflictions.

Bamboo. *(Bambusa, Dendrocalamus).* Many genera of Bamboo have been used for food for thousands of years in China. The inner portions are sweet and tender and they form an important ingredient in Chinese cooking. Bamboo is also thought to be a food useful in strengthening the "third eye."

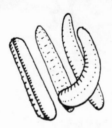

Banana *(Musa spp.).* In central Africa females believe the Banana flower can impregnate them. It is most certainly one of the most luscious, sensual flowers one could hope to see. Ralph Waldo Emerson says that where the Banana grows man is sensual and cruel. I disagree with this, as it condemns all men who live in the tropics as cruel. Banana blossoms can be sliced and added to seafood dishes, cooked as a vegetable, or served as dessert. The Bananas themselves are a perfect fruit for invalids, babes and anyone who likes fruit. Bananas contain much potassium which is sorely needed in our American diet. And if you have diarrhea the best food to eat is *ripe* Bananas—that is RIPE, as when the skin is black but the Banana starch has changed to a sugar and the flesh is mellow but without defects. It would surely be a mistake to cook Bananas, but you can do so if you like. We like to think of fruits such as the Banana and the Orange as perfect because they come in their own biodegradable wrapping which can be stripped away, thus protecting the fruit from untidy handling and potent sprays. Plantains are also a species of *Musa* which attain a larger size. They are usually eaten cooked in some way or another.

Barberry *(Berberis vulgaris)* is often grown for the fruit which can be pickled or made into jelly.

Barley *(Hordeum spp.)* seems to have preceded wheat historically as an article of the diet. It has been found in the intestinal contents of Egyptians of the pre-Dynastic periods (before 3200 B.C.). Barley was thought to have grown out of man while wheat grew out of woman. Barley is used as food, in brewing (for malt liquor), as a medicinal substance, and in cosmetics.

Basil *(Ocimum Basilicum, O. minimum)* is a sweet, wondrous-smelling plant that is so pleasant with the Tomato or the turtle. Fresh Basil is best, but if you can only get dried, try placing a drop of essential oil of Basil on several ounces of the dried herb. Toss the mixture to blend and store it away so that the oil will infuse with the herb. You can then use this dried but scented Basil as you would the fresh. Pesto is that delicious Italian sauce made with fresh Basil pounded with Olive oil, Pine nuts, Parmesan, Parsley, Garlic, salt, and Pepper. Use pesto sauce on spaghetti rings, green noodles (pasta verde), freshly sauteed Onions, spread on toasted bread, on vegetables, and in salads.

Bay Laurel leaves *(Laurus nobilis,* the Noble Bay, and the California Bay, *Umbellularia californica)* have an affinity with many diverse kinds of food. They are used dried or fresh, and with a very light hand as their volatile oils are very potent. Along with Marjoram, Thyme, and Parsley, Bay leaves make up the ubiquitous bouquet garni that is used in many meat and vegetable dishes. It is especially useful in vegetables, noodle dishes, condiments and soups. In ancient times Bay leaf was thought to be beneficial to the health and happiness of man.

Beans *(Phaseolus spp.)* I like referring to them as *flowers.* When combined with the proper *grasses,* such as Rice or Corn, beans make up perfect proteins. So remember whenever you eat a *grass,* make sure you combine it with a *flower* so that not only will you be eating carbohydrates you will, in fact, be eating proteins. Beans looked so much like testicles to the Egyptians that they revered them and forbade their use as a food. Most Beans should be soaked for some time before they are used, as this soaking breaks down zinc-binding phytate, thus releasing zinc and other vital nutrients. The long soaking starts the sprouting process which increases the amount of vitamins and proteins that will be in the Beans. And if you really want to be healthy, sprout your Beans more often, eat them raw in salads and forego the cooking; we are destroying our health with our fanaticism about cooking everything that we eat. Garlicked Beans are used to cure coughs.

Bearberry *(Arctostaphylos Uva-ursi)*. These berries have been eaten by American Indians, made into a cider, and the leaves have been used as medicine for the bladder and kidneys, for sprained backs, for poison oak, and as a smoking tobacco.

Bedstraw, Lady's *(Galium verum)* is so named because it was one of the plants thought to have been put in the Baby Jesus' manger. It also has the property of curdling milk and was used in Cheshire cheese making.

Beets *(Beta vulgaris)* are eaten and some are grown as sugar beets. The edible Beet is used in one doctor's diet as an anti-aging food. We like boiled Beets seasoned with Mint, Parsley, Tarragon, Basil, or Dill. Cold sliced Beets are good with a dressing of oil and Lemon juice. Turnips, which are a sort of white Beet, are used as a wash to remove dandruff or running sores on the head.

▲**Bergamot** *(Monarda didyma)*, also called Bee Balm or Oswego Tea, is one of the plants the colonists drank in place of India Tea at the time of the Boston Tea Party on December 16, 1773. It has both a Lemony scent and flavor. The flowers are used in salads, wine drinks or cold drinks, and the leaves are used for tea or salads.

Berries of all kinds are eaten and loved by people throughout the world. They are a food to eat fresh, ripe and uncooked. They are used in making wines, liqueurs (Black currant/cassis), condiments, desserts and salads.

[The Peach, the Apple, and the Blackberry: A Peach and an Apple once quarreled as to which was the fairer fruit. They were so loud in their discourse that a Blackberry from the next hedge overheard them. "Come," said the Blackberry, "we are all friends; pray let us have no jangling among ourselves."]

Aesop's Fables

▲**Betel** *(Areca catechu)* is a masticatory and not strictly a drug; it is the world's most used masticatory and is mildly narcotic. It is used for overacidity and in sandwiches. Betel is made from the palm seed *Areca catechu* and the leaf of *Piper Betle.*

Betony, Wood *(Betony officinalis* or *Stachy's officinalis)* is also called Bishop's wort. The flowers have a really divine smell, a sweet taste, and can be added to salads. The leaves are used in tea or in smoking mixtures. Once Betony was the sovereign remedy for any problems relating to the head, and the tea was used for asthma or varicose veins.

Blessed Thistle *(Cnicus benedictus)* has been eaten and used as a food since Roman times. The young leaves can be cut into salads and the flower heads eaten like Artichokes.

Borage *(Borago officinalis)* flowers are used in salads and drinks, and have a cucumber scent and flavor. The very young leaves can be picked and used in salads, are a traditional flavoring in the drink "Pimms No. 1 cup," and can be chopped finely into cheese. Borage is said to have a wondrous effect on the body (it feeds the adrenals) and mind; in fact, it is used to stimulate the "third eye". An ancient proverb says that Borage brings courage. Borage contains calcium and potassium.

Bouquet Garni is a combination of Thyme and Bay leaf tied with a sprig of Parsley and a string so that it can be easily removed. It is used to flavor soup and stews.

▲**Buckwheat** *(Fagopyrum esculentum)* is one of my favorite foods. We occasionally eat the groats, but it is the delicious stone-ground flour mixed with water and baked to make cakes that excites me. Top that off with Maple syrup and you have a breakfast fit for royalty. Sour-dough Buckwheat waffles just might be better.

My Uncle Ed was a fanatic for perfectly ground Buckwheat flour. Once while visiting him in Canada in the dead of an icy winter, he and I drove over slick roads to get to the market that had the perfect flour and head cheese. He baked those pancakes on his wood stove and poured on thick dark Maple syrup, freshly churned butter and ultra-thin slices of head cheese. Ah! The fragrance and warmth of that Canadian kitchen comes back to me whenever I make Buckwheat cakes.

Buckwheat contains much rutin, a bioflavonoid (Vitamin P), which increases capillary strength and regulates capillary permeability. They are companions to Vitamin C and keep "collagen, the intercellular cement, in healthy condition" (John Kirschmann, *Nutrition Almanac*, p. 59).

Burdock *(Arctium lappa)* is a large, handsome plant belonging to the Thistle group of the order *Compositae*. The stalks, boiled and stripped of the outer covering, make a tender vegetable that is also used medicinally for a beautiful complexion. These stalks, which are cut before the plant flowers, can also be thinly sliced, marinated in oil and vinegar, and eaten raw. Burdock is a traditional food of the Orient.

Burnet, Greater *(Poterium sanguisorba,* or *Sanguisorba minor,* the common or garden Burnet)* is a spring herb. It is a perennial grass that is refreshing to eat, slightly diuretic, and a minor source of Vitamin C. It can be used to make vinegars, wine and tea, and in salads. The salad Burnet *(Pimpinella saxifraga)* or lesser Burnet is used in much the same way as the greater Burnet. These plants have a Cucumber-like smell and flavor.

▲**Cacao** *(Theobroma Cacao),* the seed of the chocolate tree, is ground up, sweetened, and used extensively in desserts and drinks. Chocolate mixed with Vanilla beans was used in Montezuma's court and called *chocolatl;* this drink later came to be mixed with sugar and thought to have aphrodisiacal powers. The Aztec Indians thought that there was a divine origin to the plant, and thus it was given the name "Food of the Gods," or *Theobroma.* The typical taste and aroma of chocolate is developed by a fermentation process. Chocolate contains the stimulant caffeine and theobromine and probably should not be given to young people; try substituting carob instead.

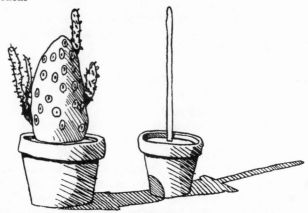

Cactus Flowers & Fruits of many species are eaten and made into various comestibles. The pulpy leaves of the nopal Cactus, called *nopales* in Mexican stores, come canned whole or diced and can be used in scrambled eggs, with onion and red chili sauce, or fried over meats such as pork chops.

Calamint *(Calamintha officinalis)* or mountain balm comes from the Greek words *"Kalos"* which means excellent, and *"mintha,"* which means mind. It has an aromatic scent and taste rather like mint and is used in teas, conserves, and in the preparation of Italian vegetables such as zucchini. "Kalos (excellent because of the ancient belief in its power to drive away serpents and the dreaded Basilisk— the fabled King of the Serpents, whose very glance was fatal.)" (Grieve, p. 153.)

▲**Calamus** *(Acorus Calamus, Calamus aromaticus)* root is candied while the leaves have been used to flavor puddings. The following information was sent to me regarding the carcinogenic properties of Calamus. In the Federal Register of May 9, 1968, 33 F. R. 6967, a study showed that when the Jammu variety of oil of Calamus was fed to rats, the rats "produced a significant number of malignant tumors of the upper small intestine. . . Chronic feeding studies are not available on other varieties of the oil of Calamus. . ."

Camomile *(Anthemis nobilis)* the Roman Camomile, is a largish, coarse perennial with flowers on a foot high stem that have a large, yellow center with white rays. *Anthemis nobilis,* the variation English mat-type perennial, is a Camomile with flowers about six inches high, yellow with no white rays. These two plants are often confused. *Matricaria Chamomilla,* Hungarian or German Camomile, is an annual with yellow flowers with white rays that grows to about a foot or more. The Roman and German Camomile have a wonderful apple-like fragrance and are used medicinally, to flavor liqueurs, in Spanish sherry, herb beers, and as a delicious soothing tea. The ancient Egyptians revered this plant for its fantastic virtues.

Capers *(Capparis spinosa)* are the flower-buds of this plant which are pickled and used in canapés, on Eggplant, eggs, fish, eel, and in steak tartare. Pickled Nasturtium buds can be used as a substitute for capers.

Capsicums are all those wonderful plants whose fruits give you green Bell Peppers, red Bell Peppers (just ripened green ones), Chiles, Paprika, Cayenne and all kinds of Peppers except, of course, the spice Pepper *(Piper). Capsicum annuum* is the most widely cultivated and probably originated in Mexico, while *C. frutescens* probably originated in South America. Archeologically, Peppers have been found in Mexican caves that date back to 7000 B.C. They are absolutely necessary in most Mexican and Indian cooking although the Chiles in hot curries were not put there until the English brought the Chiles to India in the Seventeenth Century.[1] Cayenne is used medicinally as one of the most active stimulants and is extremely useful in soups where it can act to cauterize a sore throat. Capsicums contain much Vitamin A and C. As an example, 100 grams of raw hot red Pepper contain 21,600 units of Vitamin A while 100 grams of Carrot contain a mere 11,000 units and Parsley only 8,500 units of Vitamin A. 100 grams of raw hot red Pepper contain 369 mg. of Vitamin C while the same weight of Strawberry leaves contain 229 mg. of Vitamin C, and 100 grams of freshly squeezed Orange juice contains a puny 50 mg of Vitamin C. The *C. annuum* group includes most of the sweet, fleshy Peppers and the hot little Bird Pepper, while *C. frutescens* includes most of the hot Peppers. A simple and delicious hot oil, or Red oil, can be made by filling a four ounce jar with small hot red Chiles, a couple of peeled Garlic cloves, one Star Anise, a bit of Ginger, and then adding Peanut oil to fill the remaining space. Use this oil, after it has steeped, been sealed, and refrigerated for a couple of weeks, to season cold chicken, cold noodles, or soup. "The active ingredient of highly pungent Chiles is capaicin, an aromatic phenol so potent that it is said to be detectable to the taste when present in so diluted a proportion as 1 part per million."[2]

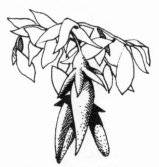

1. A note on chile peppers and their famous relative, chili. The peppers are spelt 'chile,' plural 'chiles,' while the beans and chile pepper combination is 'chili.'
2. Robert W. Schery, *Plants for Man*, p. 529 (see Bibliography).

When I think about Cayenne, I think of Jeremy Fisher and mothers who admonish their children not to get their feet wet lest they catch a cold, and this always reminds me of a passage from Beatrix Potter's book, *The Tale of Jeremy Fisher,* "But Mr. Jeremy liked getting his feet wet; nobody ever scolded him, and he never caught a cold!" Cayenne is used in socks to keep the feet warm and is placed on bare, wet feet to stimulate the circulation so that one won't catch a cold.

My father always had a dish of home-grown marinated chiles by his plate to eat with meals. It was my great desire to someday be able to eat a meal with him and match his ability to eat these nose-running, mouth-searing, eye-watering, delicious little morsels as he did. Shortly before he died and after years of practice on my part, I did indeed sit with him, converse, and eat those vitamin-packed chiles.

Caraway *(Carum Carvi)* seeds have an anise or licorice-like flavor and are used in herb breads, Mushroom sauce, salads, Asparagus, Beets, Potatoes, sauerkraut, Cabbage, cheeses, baked fruit, poultry, liqueurs (Kümmel), soups and love potions.

Cardamom *(Elettaria Cardamomum)* seeds are delicious in coffees and liqueurs, curry mixtures, breads, pastries, to flavor fruit salads, and to whiten teeth. They were originally used as an aromatic stimulative carminative.

Cardoons are related to Artichokes and Celery and are used in much the same way.

▲**Carnation** *(Dianthus Caryophyllus)* is an old-fashioned flower that makes a tasty addition to white wines. The flowers of this species as well as other *Dianthus* can be used to flavor and scent salads. The flavor is rather sweet and slightly biting, as is the scent, and they are also used to flavor wines, vinegars, cordials, syrups, marmalades, jellies and herb butters. They rejoice the senses through their scent and taste.

▲**Carob** *(Ceratonia Siliqua)*. St. John's Bread and Locust Pods are just two of the common names of this ancient plant. It was thought to clear the throat and was thus used by those who use their throats a lot (singers and clergymen). More important is its nutritious use as a substitute for Chocolate. Carob is a natural sweetener with a flavor similar to Chocolate but decidedly more rich in vitamins and minerals, and it should definitely be used by people who wish to avoid caffeine such as that found in Chocolate, Coffee and tea. Ten grams (1 T) of Carob contains one tenth the fat, half the calories and five times more calcium than an equal weight of Chocolate. So do substitute Carob for Chocolate as a treat; it is much more healthful and may even contribute to your peace of mind. Carob seeds are the original "carat" weight once used by jewelers.

Carrots *(Daucus Carota)* are one of the root vegetables that I doubt we could do without. It is used cosmetically as a cleanser, medicinally in many diets (especially those called mucousless), as a vegetable, and in jams.

▲**Cashews** *(Anacardium occidentale)* are delicious nuts that can be eaten either fresh or roasted. They are delicious in pies, granolas, and in nut mixes.

▲**Cassia** *(Cinnamomum Cassia).* See Cinnamon.

Catnip *(Nepeta Cataria)* is more famous for its use in attracting cats than in feeding people. In my garden a large round steel cage surrounds the Catnip plant to keep it safe from the marauding neighborhood "panthers". Catnip has been used to flavor meats, salads and sauces, although it is better put to use in the herbal medicine chest where it fights fever and insomnia. Catnip/Camomile tea is great for hysteria.

Cattails *(Typha spp.)* When young were eaten as a green vegetable by California Indians. In the winter the roots become filled with a starchy material and can be shredded and used as a salad or cooked as a vegetable. Cattail fluff can be used to stuff pillows or beds, especially baby beds. One of my most loved possessions is a pillow that has been stuffed with this fluff given me by my friend Nan. The pollen of this plant has also been made into bread.

Celery *(Apium graveolens)* tops are excellent added to soups, stews, in the water to cook Artichokes, in fasting drinks and teas, and in aphrodisiacal mixtures. If you are a witch, you of course know that you must eat Celery seeds before flying off for a witch festival so that you won't fall off your broom. The original wild Celery was called Smallage. Celery stalks make a delicious and healthful snack.

Chenopodiaceae is an order of plants that produces many edible seeds and leaves. Most of these plants contain iron in large quantities that can be easily digested.

Cherry *(Prunus spp.)* is a delicious fruit that has often been used in the treatment of gout and arthritis. By all means eat them raw. Cherry stems are used in diuretic teas.

Chervil *(Anthriscus Cerefolium)* is a hardy annual used as a garnish in sauces, soups, eggs, cheese, breads, salads, and fish. It has a bright green color and a mild taste that has been described as similar to Parsley with a hint of Anise. This warm spicy herb we like best generously sprinkled over cold cream soups, fresh green salads, Carrots or Potatoes. Used generously on foods it is very stimulating to the metabolism. Try seasoning peeled Avocadoes with Olive oil, Pepper, Lemon juice and a really generous dose of chopped Chervil. You will soon find that this herb is as essential in your cooking as it is to the French, who use quantities of it.

Chestnut *(Castanea spp.)* nuts are delicious and imported into the United States from Italy. They are eaten roasted, in soups, in puddings, and are about 10% protein.

Chickweed *(Stellaria Media)* is very high in the nutrients iron, calcium and copper. It can be used in salad and salad dressings as it has a soothing quality that herbalists call emollient or demulcent. It soothes irritated or inflamed tissues; it is a food to soothe and heal the digestive system as well as an herb to discourage obesity. A simple salad dressing using Chickweed can be made in a blender using a large handful of the plant, a Garlic clove or two, 1/2 cup vegetable oil, 1 Lemon juiced, a bit of Kelp, a pinch of Rosemary or Basil, and blending until smooth. Add Lemon or oil and salt to taste.

Chicory *(Cichorium Intybus)* varieties are divided into groups, root types and the others. They all contain Vitamin C and have a tonic and diuretic action on the system. Witloof (Belgian endive) is a root Chicory even though the blanched leaves rather than the root are eaten. Endive and Escarole are also Chicories and are eaten for their rather bitter leaves, while wild Chicory is eaten for the roots as well as being roasted and added to coffee.

Chile see Capsicum

Chives *(Allium Schoenoprasum)* are mildly flavored members of the Onion family and can be used as a garnish, in soups or sauces, delicious on eggs or cheese, and in any fish or vegetable recipe. They are probably most famous as an ingredient on Texas baked potatoes, that is, a crispy on the outside, soft on the inside baked Potato that has been heaped with butter, sour cream, bacon, Chives and grated Parmesan. They are also called *Ail civitte,* or Cives and Civit leaves (do not confuse them with Civet the cat). Another type of Chives are the Garlic Chives, somewhat larger and with a more pronounced fragrance and flavor.

Chlorella is a unicellular freshwater algae, a complete vegetable protein cultivated in special tanks and ponds under maximum growth conditions to give all the vitamins and minerals in a concentrated form. It is a pure natural source of quick energy, and it can also increase endurance. The chlorophyll rebuilds the hemoglobin in the blood while the body detoxifies. Try it!

Chrysanthemums of many types are used in cooking, in salads, in tea blends, in wines, in soups, poultry, and sauces. They are especially esteemed by the Japanese and Chinese. Mary MacNichol in *Flower Cookery,* p. 28 (see Bibliography), states,

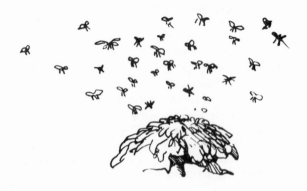

"In China it is believed that eating Chrysanthemums increases longevity, will turn white hair black again, make the body light and vigorous and after eating Chrysanthemum pills the teeth will grow again."

Cicely, Sweet *(Myrrhis odorata)* is often called sweet Chervil and Myrrh plant. It is not at all related to the gum Myrrh. Sweet Cicely is used to regulate young girls' menstrual cycles. It has been used as a salad herb and the root can be boiled as a vegetable.

Cilantro, see Coriander

Cinnamon *(Cinnamomum zeylanicum)* is the dried, fragrant bark of the Cinnamon tree. It is an ancient spice indigenous to Sri Lanka (Ceylon) and India, originally used for embalming purposes, then often used to disguise the taste and scent of rotting meat, sometimes used as an aphrodisiac, and now mainly used to flavor and scent potpourris, drinks, coffee, fruit, pickles or mutton. It acts as an aromatic stimulant.

Citron *(Citrus medica)* is an edible fruit; called Etrog it is important in Jewish tradition during the Feast of the Tabernacles. In the Middle Ages it was used as an antidote for poisons, which may have been because of its Vitamin C content. It is said that Alexander the Great introduced this fruit to the Mediterranean area about 300 B.C., and it was quite popular in Roman times. The rind is very thick and is frequently candied.

Citronnella *(Cymbopogon nardus)* is a grass sometimes called Lemon Balm and is usually used as a tea herb or in herbal mixtures, especially for drinking or for baking fish.

▲**Clary, Sage** *(Salvia Sclarea)* is a large plant originating in the Mediterranean area, introduced into England in 1562, and used in wines, food and medicine. As a substitute for Hops in beer, it is said that Clary produces an "insane exhilaration of spirits" followed by a severe headache. This beer, however, is also used in treating women's complaints and problems. Clary can be used in omelets, as fritters, or in soups.

Clivers *(Galium aparine)* seeds are sometimes roasted and used to adulterate or substitute for coffee, and the leaves are used for tea.

Clove *(Eugenia caryophyllata).* The dried flower buds are used as a spice. They are strongly pungent, chewed for bad breath (they perfumed breath in early China), used in desserts or spice cakes, for pickling, to spice wild game, ham or pork, mutton, fruits, and used in the making of potpourris and pomanders.

Clover *(Trifolium spp.)* is mainly used as fodder or in phytotherapy. Its main culinary use is to provide much nectar for bees so that they can make delicious Clover honey.

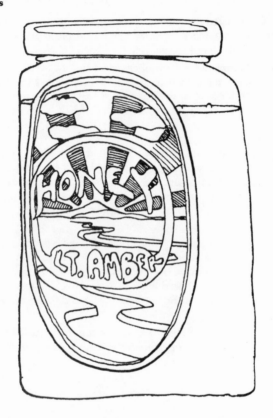

The pedigree of honey
Does not concern the bee;
A clover, any time, to him
Is aristocracy.

Emily Dickinson

Clover is used in the making of wine, sandwiches, tea, vinegar, bath mixtures, and pickled in salads. Its activity is somewhat anti-fungicidal in nature.

Coconut *(Cocos nucifera)* milk, juice, flesh, and oil are all used in cooking, especially in curries, Hawaiian food, and tropical foods. The King Coconut, called *thambili* in Sinhala, is a rare and superior variety found in Sri Lanka (Ceylon) and is believed to have valuable therapeutic properties. The water contains albumen and is thirst quenching, cool, and sweet. It is given to patients who have dehydrating diseases and is also taken by drinkers to combat the effects of too much alcohol. This liquid can be given orally or intravenously. The meat contains protein, fat, carbohydrates, vitamins, and minerals, and is prescribed for malnutrition or general debility. And, as if that were not enough, the boiled meat yields an oil that is used as a hair tonic and a substitute for cod liver oil. Ask a drunk in Sri Lanka why he drinks King Coconut juice, and he says, "It clears the head, it clears the whole system" (G. Navaratne, *San Francisco Examiner,* 22 February 1976).

▲**Coffee** *(Coffea arabica)* beans roasted, ground, and cooked make one of the most tasty brews imaginable. My husband had indigestion for two years until he stopped drinking 8 cups of Coffee per day. Excess was the problem here, not the Coffee. Doc Branson says, "Coffee squeezes the adrenals dry and the next day when you need the energy of the adrenals they have nothing to give—resistance lowers and illness strikes with difficulties like circles under the eyes." I love Coffee, the smell and taste really turn me on, but I use it moderately. One delicious cup per day of Italian roast brewed in an expresso pot is my limit. I consider Coffee a drug, a delicious drug, and so, my one cup a day has got to be the very best I can get—no hotel or restaurant Coffee for me, please! About 1600 Francis Bacon said of Turkish Coffee, it is "made of a Berry of the same name, as Black as Soot, and of a Strong Scent but not Aromatical; which they take, beaten into Powder, in Water as Hot as they can Drink it; and they take it, and sip at it in their Coffee Houses, which are like our Taverns. The Drink comforteth the Brain and Heart and helpeth Digestion." Coffee is much used in cooking. [It is also used as an enema for asthma, cancer, and other problems.] Read *Coffee* by C. & V. Schafer for 123 pages of Coffee information.

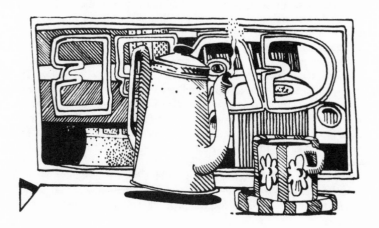

▲**Cola** *(Cola acuminata)* is used as a masticatory and as a flavoring for "Cola" drinks; it contains much caffeine and is not a suitable drink for children (especially since so much sugar is added to improve the taste), and some species are chewed as a narcotic stimulant. Approximately 100 tons of Cola are shipped to the United States from Africa annually, primarily to be used in Cola drinks, and about 150,000 tons are shipped annually to Europe. What do the Europeans do with so much cola?

Coltsfoot *(Tussilago Farfara)* is used in the making of cough drops, smoking mixtures, wine or tea, and as a useful remedy for coughs and colds.

Comfrey *(Symphytum officinala* and other *spp.)* is a most useful plant in herbal body care, herbal medicine, or in the herbal kitchen. The fresh and dried parts can be used, root or leaf. The young leaves can be chopped into salads or made into healthful green drinks. The roots can be made into teas or poultices. Comfrey can be said to be the world's fastest protein builder and is an absolute must in any vegan's diet as it is one of the few plants that can produce B12 from the cobalt in the soil. The flowers can also be added to your daily green salad that, of course, you eat every single day to be healthy, happy, and wise!

Coriander *(Coriandrum sativum)* leaves are also called Cilantro or Mexican or Japanese Parsley. They have a very specific taste and are necessary in certain foods such as guacamole, some Oriental dishes, and South American and West Indian food. The seeds are used in cheese dishes, sauces, curries, fish and lamb. Coriander was introduced to England by the Romans and has been cultivated and used since ancient times. It is used to flavor sweets, liqueurs, and to scent perfumes and potpourris.

Corn *(Zea Mays),* Maize, Seed of seeds, Sacred Mother and Giver of Life are all common names for this grass whose original home was in the Americas. If Beans can be called "flowers" and Corn "grass," then all you have to remember when you want to combine foods properly to make complete proteins is that a "grass" plus a "flower" make a perfect combination. Beans and rice, black-eyed peas and wheat, and Beans and Corn are all combinations that can be termed perfect. Corn in the Americas was the basis of some religions and a symbol of fertility. The Zunis have many folktales relating to Corn and use the different colors of Corn in their ceremonies. The cardinal points were especially important; yellow Corn was used for the north, red Corn for the south, blue Corn for the west and white Corn for the east. Blue Corn was the most popular and important to the Indians, and was used medicinally as well as for its superior taste. (Write to Roybal Store, Rear 214 Galisteo St., Santa Fe, New Mexico, 87501.) I especially like Blue Corn tortillas, and when a friend sent me twenty-five pounds of blue corn as a present, I immediately took it to La Palma Mexicatessen here in San Francisco and had it made into delicious and nutritious tortillas. You can probably find a tortilleria in your own area that will make tortillas for you out of blue Corn. Blue Corn has to be cooked with an alkaline substance like juniper ashes or baking powder or else the Corn turns purple when it bakes. Delicious blue corn pancakes can be made with 2−3 cups of fine blue Cornmeal, 1 cup of Whole Wheat pastry flour, an optional teaspoonful of baking powder, and enough milk or goat milk to make a pancake batter. Cook the pancakes on a hot griddle greased with Corn oil and serve with sweet butter and Maple syrup. Although not quite a 100% Indian meal, it definitely is an American delight. These cakes can also be served with beans sandwiched between and red Chile sauce on top.

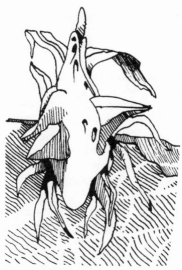

Costmary *(Chrysanthemum Balsamita)* leaves can be chopped up and used as a minty flavor in salads. The scent is ever so slightly repulsive to me so I do not use it, which is not to say that it should not be used. It is also used in soups, eggs, meat and drinks.

Cowslips and Primrose *(Primula veris)* has been used since ancient times to strengthen the nerves and soothe the mind. Its flowers are yellow and fragrant and used in salads, syrups, vinegars, wine, pickles, and can be candied.

Cranberry *(Vaccinium oxycoccus* and *V. macrocarpon).* These berries are good for kidney infections. One to two cups of the boiled juice should be taken by those prone to recurring kidney infections or stones.

Cubebs *(Piper Cubeba)* are the dried, unripe fruits of the plant which are used in cookery, and which act medicinally as a stimulant.

Cucumber *(Cucumis sativus)* is a cooling plant that is best eaten raw with a sprinkle of dill weed or Chervil, although it can be made into the most delicious iced soup with yogurt. (See *The Herbal Body Book* for many cosmetic formulas.)

Cumin *(Cuminum Cyminum)* is an annual plant whose taste definitely reminds me of Mexican food. Whenever I smell it, my mouth immediately begins to salivate and I can just taste delicious tortillas with sauces, Beans and Chiles.

When I was researching the chapter on Aromatherapy in *The Herbal Body Book,* I was also nursing a two-month-old baby boy. He and I spent many hours together inhaling the odors of many fragrant plants. Whenever he smelled Jasmine he would go to sleep, whenever he smelled Carrot seed oil he would cry, but whenever he smelled Cumin oil he would lay back, smile and poop. I still haven't figured out exactly what this means. Cumin is much used to season cheeses and a whole host of other dishes from Cabbage to eggs to meats.

Curry Plant *(Helichrysum angustifolium)* is a plant that does not furnish the seasoning Curry. Curry seasoning is made up of anywhere from five to twenty-five different herbs and spices. The Curry plant, however, has the pungent scent of Curry in its leaves which are used in preparing chicken, eggs, and salads.

Daisy *(Bellis perennis),* also called Bruisewort, flowers from the earliest days of spring and covers the ground closely. It is used in lawns for an English countryside effect. In former days, the Daisy was sometimes used as a potherb, although the leaves are rather bitter. It is most often used as a decoction externally to soothe overexercised muscles.

Dandelion *(Taraxacum officinale)* is one of Mother Nature's most important healing agents. It is a specific for the liver and, being partly French, I feel that the liver is the most important body organ. If you have a healthy liver, you will have a healthy body. So we use Dandelion as a bitter green in all our spring salads. At New Age Creations Dandelion is used along with Comfrey in over ninety of the herbal mixtures. Dandelion greens contain large amounts of Vitamins A and C, and minerals such as potassium, calcium, manganese, and sulphur. It is an extremely agreeable plant and can be eaten raw, in teas, or as a potherb. The root is used medicinally as a diuretic and can be roasted as a substitute for coffee. Dandelion flowers are used in the making of wine.

Dill *(Anethum graveolens)* is a popular culinary plant whose dried ripe fruit has a long history of use both as a medicinal and a kitchen herb. Dill is delicious on small boiled Potatoes and little Carrots, and, of course, is a necessity in Dill pickles. Dill seed soaked in milk is used to cure flatulence, especially in children, and will soothe a restless infant to sleep. Dill leaves are a tasty wrapping to whole baked fish.

Dittany of Crete *(Origanum Dictamnus)* leaves mixed with Parsley, Garlic, Thyme, salt, and Pepper make an interesting fish sauce. The leaves can also be chewed for a sore throat.

Dock *(Rumex spp.)* grows abundantly in my backyard, and, although it comes very near the top of the list for Vitamin C and A content, its taste is just a bit too coarse and rambunctious for me to use this plant in my kitchen. So we use Dock mainly as a medicinal with Comfrey and plantain. These are old plants and have been used as potherbs and written about for several thousand years.

Eggplant *(Solanum Melongena)* actively aids the excretion of bile and is delicious to eat.

Elder *(Sambucus nigra)* has wonderful properties that make it essential in the cosmetic chest and extremely useful in the kitchen. It has been used in cooking, baking, wine and liqueur making. All parts of the tree are used: leaves, flowers, berries, and bark. A standard cure for the flu is an infusion of Elder flowers and Peppermint. The berries are used for making pies and sweets, and to color port. The plant has so many folk uses that it would take many pages to describe them, but Charles Skinner, in his *Myths and Legends* (see Bibliography), has said it nicely: "Elder wood cures toothache, keeps the house from attack, fends off snakes, mosquitoes, and warts, quiets nerves, interrupts fits, removes poisons from metal vessels, keeps worms out of furniture, and guarantees that he who cultivates it shall die in his own house." An Italian liqueur called *Sambuca Romana* is made from the Elder berries and leaves.

Elecampane *(Inula helenium)* is a potent medicinal plant used for thousands of years. It is used chiefly for coughs and respiratory complaints. The root has been candied and eaten as a sweetmeat.

Elm, Slippery *(Ulmus fulva)* bark has a rather slimy, mucilaginous taste, and mixed with Lemon juice, Licorice syrup and water is used as a food to cure bowel infections such as dysentery and diarrhea. This tree is indigenous to North America and the knowledge of its wonderful strengthening and healing qualities was given to white men by the Indians.

Epazote *(Chenopodium ambrosioides)* is the Mexican herb par excellence. It is commonly known as Mexican tea or wormseed. It reduces the gassiness you get from eating Beans. Mexican or Cuban black Beans cannot be properly cooked without a sprig of Epazote.

Fennel *(Foeniculum vulgare,* for the seeds; *F. dulce,* also called Florence Fennel, for the root). An absolutely fantastic number one remedy for *everything,* especially any problems relating to the eyes, is a decoction of Fennel seed and comfrey root cooled, strained, and refrigerated for use. Always have it on hand. This mixture can be used externally or internally; it is truly fantastic, being soothing, healing, and cleansing. Fennel seeds are also used to sweeten milk for indigestion, in soups, for fish, in liqueurs, in cookies, in vegetables and salads, and for poultry and game. Fennel stalks wrapped around fish to be roasted is delicious. The sliced root is delicious eaten raw as part of a vegetable salad, or marinated in Olive oil and

Lemon juice, salt and Pepper. It has digestive qualities that reduce the oiliness in foods and is especially useful in reducing diets.

Fenugreek *(Trigonella Foenum-graecum)* seeds and sprouts contain iron and Vitamin B12 in a form that one can assimilate; they are delicious, and especially recommended for diabetics. Everyone should add this herb to the daily salad. It is a kind of legume (a flower in my protein terminology), and should be combined with a grass (such as Corn or Wheat) to make a complete protein.

Ferns of many species are used cosmetically and medicinally. The tightly curled ends of the fronds of some common Ferns when they just emerge from the soil are called fiddleheads, and are eaten somewhat the same way as one would eat Asparagus. They can be toxic, however, if eaten over a long period of time and can interfere with metabolism.

Figs *(Ficus carica)*. The Fig tree has many legends associated with it. The leaves provided Adam and Eve with a covering to hide their nakedness and the fruit itself is thought by some to have been the fruit of knowledge that caused this first couple such trouble (and us too for that matter). Both the Christians and the Jews have associated this tree with lust and fertility. The ancient Greeks fed on nothing but Figs to increase strength and speed. It is interesting that the Fig is neither fruit nor flower, but is a hollow receptacle filled with undeveloped flowers that never fully mature but develop mature seeds just the same. This is a succulent fruit that is best eaten out of hand.

Fines Herbes is a mixture of equal quantities of finely chopped fresh or rubbed dry herbs. The mix usually includes Chives, Parsley, Tarragon and Bay leaves. This mixture is traditionally French and is used in egg dishes, salads, sauces, and also fish and poultry.

Fir tree needles have been employed in cookery, especially as an addition to game such as venison and rabbit, in lamb stew, or with beef stock.

Flowers of many kinds are used in cookery, in sauces, in salads. When I speak of *flowers* and *grasses* as being protein complements I mean that the flowers which represent legumes (Beans and Peas) complement the protein in the seed heads of grasses (Corn, Wheat and Rice). And so to eat economical and healthy proteins one must eat a combination of flowers and grasses.

Fruits of all kinds are eaten. They are of much use during fasting diets or for cleansing diets. Fruits definitely should be eaten uncooked to be of the most value. The flowers of fruits are used in syrups, salads, and teas.

Fuchsia is named after the great German botanist, Leonard Fuchs, who included this lovely flower in his book of woodcuts. It is easily grown and was used by the California Indians for contusion types of injuries. The ripe fruit makes a delicious jam, pie, or sauce.

Fungi (mushrooms, etc.) of many kinds are eaten and enjoyed. The magical drink of the Hindu Gods, called *Soma,* is now thought to be derived from *Amanita muscaria,* that lovely mushroom with a festive red and white dress. Once when I was teaching in Mendocino, I used it as an example of a plant that had been thought deadly but could in fact be used in moderation in various ritualistic ceremonies. Many of the people in the room had never seen an Amanita, and so it was passed around. When it finally got back to me, only the stalk was left. It seemed that my lovely Amanita had been devoured by seekers of *Soma* as it had made its way around the room.

Garlic *(Allium sativum).* What can I say about this fabulous bulb that has not already been said? It is tasty, delicious, antibacterial, antifungal and absolutely necessary in all kinds of cooking. There is one definitive Garlic book entitled *The Book of Garlic, The Incredible Story of Allium Sativum as Magic Bulb, Potent Medicine, Unrivalled Culinary Herb and Stinking Rose of Mirth,* by Lloyd J. Harris. If you want this book or want to find out about a very select club called "Lovers of the Stinking Rose," write to him at 1043 Cragmont Ave., Berkeley, CA 94708.

Geranium *(Pelargonium spp.)* plants, the scented leaved varieties, make up a large portion of my yard. In the early summer when the plants are blooming, the flowers are picked regularly and used in the making of moist potpourris, or simply dropped into flower salads. The leaves are picked and used in salad dressings, drinks, soups, scented butters and on vegetables such as Cauliflower. There are many scents and flavors to the scented-leaved Geraniums, so select leaves with the specific taste and fragrance that will best complement the food you are serving.

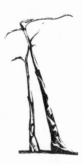

Ginger *(Zingiber officinale)* root is used in curry powders, pickles, Eastern foods, pastries, soups, cheese, and stews. It has a fine aromatic scent and a spicy, hot taste. Ginger prefers to grow in a hot humid climate with heavy rainfall, and you can provide this type of environment in the bathroom where it makes an attractive house plant. Ginger infused in yogurt will stimulate digestion and ease flatulence. It also has antiseptic qualities that make it useful as a digestive.

Ginseng *(Panax quinquefolius* or *P. schinseng)* nourishes the creative part of a person, clears perception, and energizes the body when taken in small amounts over a long period of time. At the time of this writing, 1977, very good quality Ginseng was selling for $30−35 per pound. Although *not* the most expensive herb in the world, it *is* one of the most useful. Like bee pollen, Ginseng can help people who are under a lot of stress. Ginseng is under the influence of the planet Saturn and under the sign of Capricorn. Ginseng can best be used in tea form, by chewing a piece, or in tonic or extract form. A ginseng liqueur can be made by macerating a Ginseng root in any liquor of your choice, such as *Sambuca Romana* or vodka. Do not take Ginseng with Vitamin C or acid drinks.

Gladiolus *(Gladiolus spp.)* is a common garden flower native to South Africa whose name means "little sword" because of the leaf shape. The flowers are eaten in salads or used as an edible boat container for various stuffings. They can also be used in sauces, omelets, potato dishes, and seem to work well with Corn and Beans.

Good-King-Henry *(Chenopodium Bonus-Henricus)* like the other members of the Chenopodium order, or goosefoots, contain organic iron in a digestible form. Good-King-Henry was once cultivated in all English gardens and used extensively as a potherb. The common names are English Mercury and All Good.

Gotu Kola *(Hydrocotyl asiatica minor)* is a marsh Pennywort that I have seen growing abundantly on the island of Maui. It is an easy plant to cultivate; it needs a moist acid soil (the addition of Pine needles works well as a mulch), some shade and a moderate humidity. Gotu Kola and Fo-Ti-Tieng are *not* the same plant, even though you will often find two such labeled jars side by side on herb store shelves. Actually, Fo-Ti-Tieng is not an individual plant at all; it is a copyrighted herbal blend of the Hindu variety of Gotu kola, Cola nut and Meadowsweet. It is available from Kev Enterprises, P. O. Box 226, Honolulu, Hawaii, 96810. Gotu kola leaves can be added to salads or they can be used as a tea; I prefer to just pick a leaf or two every day and eat them.

Grapevine *(Vitis vinifera).* Grapes have been grown for many thousands of years. The leaves are used in cooking, and the fruit! What could I say in a little paragraph that could possibly do justice to wine? My father grew Grapes and made raisins and always as a girl I had one or another of these to eat. It wasn't until I went away to college that I realized that other folks got their Grapes and raisins at stores. My dad grew a variety of lovely seedless Grapes which were as long as your little finger and so sweet; a small bunch would totally satisfy the most extravagent taste. Oh my, how I miss those home-grown treats.

Grasses. The three most important cereal foods of the world are the ripe seed heads of Wheat, Rice, and Corn. (See also flowers.)

Guarana *(Paullinia cupana)* contains more caffeine than do coffee or tea (5%), and much more tannin (5%). Brewed with water, like coffee, and with sugar added, it makes a very potent and stimulating beverage. It can also be taken in gelatin capsules.

▲ **Heather** *(Erica vulgaris)* makes the most divine honey. I like to eat it "straight" out of the jar, but mixed with butter and spread on graham crackers is also not bad. Heather oil from the flowers is used externally and has a reputation for curing cutaneous eruptions.

Hibiscus *(Hibiscus sabdariffa* and other *Hibiscus spp.)* flowers can be made into tasty, rather tart drinks, juices, sauces and punches.

Hollyhock *(Althaea rosea)* flowers are generally employed medicinally for their diuretic and soothing qualities, but they can be used in salads, herbal tea mixtures, or as a potherb, as they were used in China.

▲ **Honeysuckle** *(Lonicera caprifolium)* flowers have a delicious nectar that the hummingbirds and I like to suck. The flowers can be dropped into salads.

▲ **Hops** *(Humulus lupulus)* used commercially are the dried inflorescence of the female plants. The Hops plant has been in use at least since Roman times, and now is mainly used in the brewing of beer. Modern tests show that an extract of hops has antibacterial properties.

▲ **Horseradish** *(Cochlearia armoracia, Armoracia rusticana* or *A. lapathifolia)* is a perennial plant with huge leaves and a large taproot. It is best used fresh as it loses flavor when cooked. It is used in condiments, vinegars, roasts, eggs, oily fish, rich meats, salads, and is taken medicinally to stimulate the appetite and improve liver function. Try grating fresh horseradish into plain yogurt for a digestive, or apply this concoction externally for a muddy complexion, acne, or pimples. Horseradish, along with Nettle, Coriander, Horehound and Lettuce is one of the five Bitter Herbs the Jews eat during the Passover.

Hyssop *(Hyssopus officinalis)* is an ancient plant, having been used medicinally and in culinary service for centuries. It has a rather bitter, minty taste; the flowers are a useful addition to salads and cold dishes, and the leaf can be used in soups, salads, with Carrots, Mushrooms, and on meats. The name Hyssop is of Greek origin and comes from the word *azob* (a holy herb) because it was used in the cleansing of holy places. Hyssop is of great value in aiding fat digestion, and should be used with fatty meat or fish dishes. Hyssop soup made with an Onion stalk is an excellent digestive after a heavy meal.

▲ **Jasmine** *(Jasminum spp.)* fruits are often poisonous. One species of Jasmine is the most expensive herb sold in the world. Some Jasmines are picked and used for their fragrance, and Chinese Jasmine flowers are used to scent teas. Most flowers of Jasmine can be used in teas, salads, or in the making of jelly. Petal jellies, such as Jasmine Petal Jelly or Orange Petal Jelly, are generally produced in France, imported here and can be purchased in the gourmet section of large department stores. You can make flower jellies simply by following a recipe for Apple jelly and adding, before bottling, as many of the clean dry flowers as it takes to flavor. Jasmine petals can also be used to make wine, liqueur, cakes, syrups or candies.

▲**Jonquil** *(Narcissus Jonquilla)* in the language of flowers means, "I desire a return of affection." Jonquils are deliciously sweet-smelling flowers that can be candied or made into conserves. They are too big to be used in salads.

Jujube *(Zizyphus Jujuba, Z. vulgaris)* is a small plant long cultivated in China and adapted to the Mediterranean climate. The berries are eaten fresh, candied, and dried; the pit is eaten as a nut. Yes, folks, there really is a Jujube tree and those funny little candies you find at the movies are just a poor imitation of the real thing. Jujubes are used in Chinese herbal medicine for nutritive, demulcent, and pectoral purposes. M. Grieve says that "Z. lotos is thought to have been one of the sources of the famous sweet fruits from which the ancient Lotophagi [Lotus-Eaters] took their name, the liqueur prepared from which caused those who partook of it to forget even their native countries in its enjoyment."

Juniper *(Juniperus communis)* is a cone-bearing tree with an intensely aromatic odor. Only the berries are used in cooking, and they are generally used to flavour game or gin. Juniper oil and berries have medicinal uses, especially externally; they are also good to take as a preventative to sickness when going from one location to another. Juniper is a magical plant which has been used to ward off evil spirits and to repel noxious demons.

Kava Kava *(Piper methysticum)* is the famous drug plant of the South Sea Islands. The root is chewed, spat into a bowl, water added, allowed to ferment, squeezed through cloth, and then drunk. Kava is a cerebral depressant and has been used as a tea herb in aphrodisiacal as well as soporific herbal blends.

Kelp (a general name for the large brown seaweeds) contains alginic acid which combines with metallic elements in the intestines to form insoluble salts which can then be excreted from the body. Lead enters our bodies from the polluted environment (water, air, food) in which we live, and children, for instance, have been known to eat lead-based paint. If you regularly eat Seaweed or Kelp, the lead will combine with the alginic acid to form lead alginate which can be excreted. Oriental peoples who eat large amounts of sea vegetables are known to have more immunity to certain diseases that are prevalent in the western world (see also sea vegetables).

Kola Nuts *(Cola nitida* and other *spp.).* See Cola.

(Lachanthes tinctoria) also called Red Root, is indigenous to the United States; the root was used by the Seminole Indians as an invigorating tonic said to "cause brilliancy and fearless expression of the eye and countenance, a boldness and fluency of speech, and other symptoms of heroic bearing, with, of course, the natural opposite after-effects" (Millspaugh, *American Medicinal Plants,* p. 688).

Lady's-Smock *(Cardamine pratensis),* also called Bittercress or Cuckooflower, is used raw in salads to promote digestion, steamed as a potherb, or added to soups.

Lavender *(Lavandula spp.)* is a plant with an intense aromatic camphoraceous odor. Do you remember your childhood and the story of Peter Rabbit? "Old Mrs. Rabbit was a widow. She also sold herbs, and Rosemary tea, and rabbit-tobacco" (which is what we call Lavender). This points out the use of Lavender as a smoking herb as well as one we use medicinally, and of course cosmetically; for a discussion of these uses see *Herbs & Things* and *The Herbal Body Book.* Have we not all heard of Lavender water as an aftershave astringent; who can smell fresh Lavender and not think of mother or grandmother's linen closet refreshed with this aromatic herb? Never be flamboyant with Lavender in cooking until you have got the measure of its effect on different foods. The flowers can be used in punches, gin drinks, sugars, or in herbal tea blends; the flowers and leaves are useful additions to salads, dressings, stews, soups, lamb or pork roasts, in baking chicken, and making wine. Add a sprig or two to the jar when making jelly.

Lavender Cotton *(Santolina chamaecyparissus)* is an attractive shrub originally grown for medicinal and culinary purposes. It has a rather distinctive flavor and is used for fatty foods like pork, or to add flavor to stocks or seafoods.

Lemon *(Citrus Limon)* originated in Syria, is much used in cookery, and has important medicinal and cosmetic uses. Candied Lemon peel is easily made and preferred when making fruitcakes. Simply boil up the peel in sugar syrup and then let it dry in the air until the sugar crystallizes. We use Lemon in juice, soup, stew, when cooking Artichokes, squeezed on fruits and vegetables to keep them from turning brown, when broiling meat or fish, as a morning drink, and in punches and mixed drinks. Lemon flowers are a tasty and fragrant addition to punches, salads, tarts, and ice cream.

Lemongrass *(Cymbopogon citratus)* is an herb much used in tea blends. Many years ago when I first became interested in phytotherapy, this herb was extremely difficult to get, and sold for over $15.00 per pound. Now, of course, the price has been drastically reduced and the plant is easily available. It is used in fish cookery, herb vinegars and salad dressings, or wherever a robust Lemon flavor is desired. Lemongrass oil is extracted for its high Vitamin A content; most vegetarian capsules of Vitamin A are composed of this oil.

Lemon Verbena *(Lippia citriodora),* called Cédron in Mexico, is used as a tea for its mild soothing effect on the stomach and slight soporific effect on the brain. Add it fresh to fruit drinks, champagne, and lay it on top of chicken or pork and then bake as usual. It adds a very refreshing and unusual taste to food, and is used in the cooking of India, France, Mexico and South America.

Lentils *(Lens esculenta)* is one of the oldest and the most nutritious of the legumes (flowers). The seed contains about 25% protein and they are very economical to eat. Waverly Root says, "It must be admitted that lentils, left to their own devices, are a trifle monotonous in flavor. One would not want to eat them as often as beans, for instance. But their very neutrality leaves room for the use of subtle seasonings and the creation of harmonious combinations which can result in memorable dishes."*

▲**Licorice** *(Glycyrrhiza glabra)* is a member of the Legume family, as is Fenugreek. It has an intensely sweet taste that satisfies thirst rather than causing thirst. It contains precurser hormones that are useful when given to women going through menopause. It has been in continuous use since ancient Egyptian and Chinese times, and has been mentioned as their ancient Materia Medicas. The flavor is mainly used in sweets and cough drops, and to sweeten and disguise the taste of bitter medicinals.

▲**Lilac** *(Syringa vulgaris):* The First Emotions of Love. In days past when one wanted to convey a message to a friend or lover without using words, messages were composed of flowers in a manner that was both subtle and heartfelt. If you wished to break your engagement, you would send a bunch of purple Lilacs that conveyed this message. The origin of the Lilac is most interesting. It has been said that an English nobleman ruined a trusting maiden and caused her death of a broken heart. Overcome with remorse, he had a clump of Lilacs planted on her grave; those who saw them said that the flowers were white in the dawn before the sun rose, and turned purple in the first rays of the sun's light. I haven't been up early enough to see if they are white, but I do know that to find a Lilac blossom with five instead of four lobes means good luck.

    To make Lilac crystals, take small bunches of the blossoms and dip them in a gum Arabic (gum Acacia) mixture of 1 oz. gum to 1/2 cup of hot water. Let the bunches dry. Meanwhile mix 1 cup sugar, 1/2 cup water and 1 T. corn syrup, and cook it to the soft ball stage. Dip the dry bunches into this mixture, sprinkle them lightly with granulated sugar, and let them dry.

Lilies *(Lilium spp.).* All flowers of this genus are edible and are frequently used in the cuisine of the Orient. Tiger Lilies are used in Szechuan cuisine such as in *Mu Shu* pork. The flowers can be used in soups, stews, with chicken or duck, with rice or potatoes, steamed with sole, steeped in honey or vinegar, or simply dipped into batter and eaten as a fritter. Madonna Lilies were formed from the milk of Hera as it fell to earth while she suckled Hercules in her sleep.

Linden *(Tilia Europaea)* leaves and flowers make a delicious tisane that is useful at night if you have trouble sleeping. This Lime flower tea is a noted thirst quencher,

*Los Angeles Times, Feb. 10, 1977.

the honey is quite delicious and most desired, and wine and conserves can be made from the blossoms.

Lotus *(Nymphaea lutea)*. All parts of the plant are edible, especially in Chinese cuisine. The sliced tubers are especially good in soups and vegetable dishes. This is one of the plants most associated with Egypt; it occurs constantly in its art and architecture. The petals close at night and reopen in the sun, and so the flower has come to symbolize the sun and the eternal resurgence of life. It also symbolizes purity.

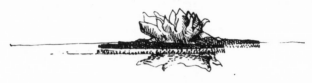

Lovage *(Levisticum officinale)* is a tall perennial herb that looks like a giant Celery and tastes like one. The flavor is quite strong. All parts of the plant can be used: leaves, stalk, seeds and root (wherever you might use Celery). This plant was formerly planted in all gardens because of its remarkable cleansing effect on the entire digestion system. We like it especially well in soups, salads, rubbed over meat, to season sauces and eggs, as a sauce for game hens, or in tea mixtures.

Mace (see Nutmeg).

Maguey or Century plant is a variety of *Agave* whose juice is extracted, fermented and distilled to form the liquor Mezcal. A maguey worm is dropped into each bottle to authenticate it. The liquor is thought to be good for the head and to act as an aphrodisiac. (Tequila comes from another Agave called the blue Agave.)

Mallow (see Marshmallow and Hollyhock). Mallows are any plants of the order Malvaceae. They are all soothing and demulcent and have edible leaves and flowers that can be used in soups, as potherbs in syrups, teas or wine. Eaten in the morning it is said to protect one from disease all day.

Manioc *(Manihot esculenta)*. The Yuca or Cassava is a much cultivated food plant. It is the staff of life to millions of people in this world. It furnishes the starch tapioca which is so delicious, as well as the foodstuff called *farinha* in Brazil. This plant has been found in archeological sites in Peru as early as 800 B.C.

Maple *(Acer saccharum)* furnishes that delicious sap that is boiled down into Maple syrup, which is an extremely important coating on buckwheat pancakes. It can also be used to glaze a ham, or in baking. It takes about 40 gallons of sap to make 1 gallon of Maple syrup. I use Maple cooking syrup and get it from the Swayzes, Brookside Farm, Tunbridge, Vermont, 05077. They use no sprays, artificial defoamers or preservatives in their syrup making.

Marigold *(Calendula officinalis)* has long been cultivated in the medicinal garden as well as the kitchen garden. The leaves were dried for broth, and were said to comfort both mind and spirit. And how could a marrow soup stock be made without the addition of these flower petals for their taste and colour? They also serve as a substitute for Saffron in rice, and will make a very different tasting bouillabaise when used in that fish stew. The leaves can be added to salads, and the petals to teas. Try scrambling eggs with Marigold, or using it in wine, pudding, or buns. It is a plant that causes no allergic reactions, and when mixed with Comfrey and Camomile is extremely useful as an internal or external application for anything. Anyone who is sensitive to plants, especially babies, will benefit from this mixture. A marigold sandwich can be made by spreading thinly sliced whole wheat bread with mayonnaise, thin slices of cheddar cheese and liverwurst, topped by fresh marigold petals and sprinkled with sesame salt (adapted from *Flower Cookery* by Mary MacNicol, p. 107).

Marjoram & Oregano are both of the genus *Origanum*. Oregano has a slightly stronger flavor than Marjoram, and so take that into account when you choose to use one of these plants on your food. Oregano is indispensable in Greek and Italian cooking, and Marjoram in French. They are used to garnish, in condiments, in soups and salads, eggs, cheese, vegetables, meat or poultry, stuffings, pasta, breads and drinks. They are especially good in Tomato dishes, Green beans, and with the plants of species *Brassica oleracea* (Brussels sprouts, Broccoli, Cabbage, Cauliflower, etc). Spaghetti is enlivened with Oregano, and Marjoram is good in Lemon soup or Mushrooms. These plants were used extensively by the ancient Romans and were used extravagantly in cooking, as they have disinfectant and preservative properties.

Marshmallow *(Althaea officinalis)* is best known for having given its name to that sticky gooey round white thing that children roast over the campfire. Originally Marshmallows were a cure for a sore chest made from the mucilage of Marshmallowroot, eggs, and sugar. Now, of course, the Mallow part has been removed, and

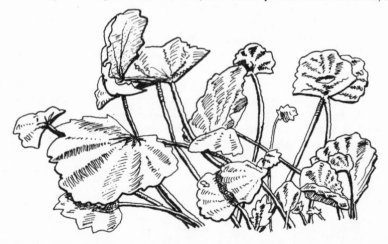

Marshmallows are simply a health-robbing confection made of sugar and little else. Mallows are softening and healing; the tops can be eaten in soup and salads, the flowers are nice in salads or to decorate raw vegetables, and root infusions are good for the urinary tract or to soothe the intestines.

▲**Maté** (see Yerba Maté).

Meadowsweet *(Spiraea ulmaria),* Queen of the Meadows, is a common wild plant that belongs to the Rose family; in olden days it was one of the favorite of the strewing herbs, and is one of the three most sacred herbs of the Druids, along with Watermint and Vervain. Meadowsweet is used in beer or wine for its slight astringency that is mildly diuretic.

Melilot *(Melilotus officinalis),* also called sweet Clover, is rather haylike in odor, and is in fact called the Mayflower. It is used to flavor cheese such as gruyère, and, put in the bath with a feverish child, will help to reduce the fever. It can also be used in stews or with rabbit. Melilot is one of the many plants that contain coumarin, an anti-coagulant that occurs in many other plants such as woodruff, tonka beans.

Melons (of the order *Cucurbitaceae*). *Cucumis spp.* gives us Melons, cantaloups and cucumbers, and *Citrullus* gives us Watermelons. They are all rather juicy fruits of edible flowers. Most Melons are mostly water; the rind is made into pickles, beer from the juice, the seeds roasted and salted are delicious as a snack, and the flesh itself, oh yummy, contains Vitamins A and C, some iron and calcium, and is, of course, a great thirst quencher.

"The watermelon is . . . chief of this world's . . . luxuries, king by grace of God over all fruits of the earth. When one has tasted it, he knows what the angels eat." (Mark Twain, *Pudd'nhead Wilson*).

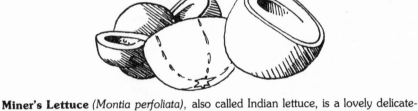

Miner's Lettuce *(Montia perfoliata),* also called Indian lettuce, is a lovely delicate-looking plant with saucer-like succulent leaves. The Indians of Placer county would gather the plant and lay it in the entrance of a red ant nest. The ants would swarm over the plants leaving a trail of formic acid which has a pleasant sour taste similar to greens dressed in vinegar. Sauté Miner's lettuce and Spinach in a bit of oil and soy sauce, or simply eat it mixed with other spring greens as a salad. It has a slight laxative effect, and was used in the spring to refresh the body after a winter of eating dried foods.

Mint *(Mentha spp.)*. There are many species of this plant and all can be eaten. They are delightfully scented aromatic hardy perennials that can be used to flavor medicine, scent the bath, or flavor foods in the kitchen. Spearmint or White Mint is especially useful in jellies or with lamb; Applemint can be used to scent and flavor salads; Pineapple Mint, Ginger Mint and Peppermint can all be used in teas or to flavor drinks, desserts or fruits. In general, Mints are good in drinks, breads, stuffings, vegetables (Eggplant, Cabbage, Lentils, Potatoes, Spinach, Mushrooms or Peas), soups, eggs, salads (Cucumber and green), meats, game, sauces or condiments. Mints are also used frequently in toothpastes, chocolate and chewing gum. Peppermint is best known for its menthol content, and is rather too strongly flavored for foods, but works well in tea mixtures, especially to settle the stomach after vomiting, in liqueurs, and as an aromatic addition anywhere where a "cooling" effect is needed.

Mintho was a nymph beloved by Pluto. Pluto's wife Proserpine was very jealous of the attention that Pluto bestowed on Mintho and so she revenged herself by turning Mintho into a lowly herb. Mintho lost her womanly beauty, but was still attractive through her refreshing fragrance.

▲**Mugwort** *(Artemisia vulgaris)*, besides being useful to give you dreams of future things, will also give you protection from evil possession when worn on St. John's Eve, June 23, and will preserve you from fatigue when put into your shoes. In addition to all this, mugwort is used in stuffing greasy poultry such as goose. The leaves are also used in moxibustion.

▲**Mulberry** *(Morus nigra)* berries are delicious eaten fresh, cooked into a pie, served with pears or other fresh fruit and cream, or juiced, jellied or jammed. Because the mulberry is dedicated to Minerva, it is considered the wisest of all the trees.

Mullein *(Verbascum Thapsis)* was thought to have the power to drive away evil spirits; a flower conserve is used to cure ringworm; the flowers in olive oil are a sovereign remedy for ear infections; the flowers add a sweet taste to salads which are eaten by asthmatics for their curative effects; the flowers soaked in milk will soothe a stomachache. One very interesting historical note is that the large woolly leaves were once used by Victorian ladies in their socks to keep their feet warm. Quite an array of interesting uses, don't you think?

Musk Seed (see Ambrette).

Mustard *(Brassica alba,* White Mustard; *B. nigra,* Black Mustard). The White Mustard is used internally and the Black, which is the more pungent, is used externally. Both are aromatic stimulants and are used prophylactically as counterirritants (who can forget the ubiquitous Mustard plaster of other days). White Mustard seeds are used in pickling, preserving and garnishing; the leaves are used in salads or in sandwiches. The Black Mustard seed makes a potent sandwich spread or a stimulating footbath.

Nasturtium *(Tropaeolum majus)*. This familiar plant is a native of Peru and was introduced into Europe in the late sixteen-hundreds. Originally adopted for its attractive flowers, Europeans later came to accept it in the kitchen also. Ancient Peruvians ate quantities of the plant, using it as a natural antibiotic to ward off infection. (Could this be related to the large quantity of Vitamin C that the plant contains?) All parts of the plant, leaves, flowers and seedpods, are edible. The plant has a rather peppery sweet taste, and it can be added to salads. Decorate salads with the flowers or fill them with cream cheese; chop flowers and add to salads or use to garnish vegetables; substitute the seedpods for Capers, or sauté them in butter and use over vegetables; mash seedpods, mix them with yogurt and mayonnaise and use over Artichokes; chop leaves and sprinkle over soups and salads. The only drawback to the Nasturtium as far as I can see is that snails also adore the plant and leave their slimy trails everywhere on it.

Nettles *(Urtica dioica* and *U. urens)* are a good spring food and may be gathered with gloves, washed, cooked in an enamel pot about 10−20 minutes, rubbed through a sieve, and then served with Pepper and a bit of butter. Their itchy stings are destroyed by drying or boiling. They are loaded with iron in a digestible form, Vitamins A and C, and nitrogen, which is both useful to the human who eats the nettle and also to the plants that get the nettles as compost. Nettles are used as blood purifiers, in reducing diets where salt should be reduced, and as a hair tonic.

Nutmeg & Mace *(Myristica fragrans)*. Mace is the net-like covering on the Nutmeg which is the fruit of the Nutmeg tree. Mace is used in pastries and biscuits, and where a strongly aromatic Nutmeg flavor is desired. The Nutmeg has a sweet, warm, and spicy taste and fragrance, and is not quite so pungent as Mace. Both are used in sauces, meats, vegetables, pastries and puddings. The Nutmeg also finds use sprinkled over drinks such as Chocolate and Coffee. Medicinally, both are intestinal stimulants.

Oats *(Avena sativa)* are among the most widely grown cereals of North America and Europe, and although they are mostly used as animal food, they are used medicinally and cosmetically as well (see *The Herbal Body Book)*. There are both spring and winter type Oats (like wheat); Oats are rich in protein but should be combined to form a complete protein (see Beans and Corn). Oats were introduced into North America in 1602, and now the United States produces most of the world's Oats.

Okra *(Hibiscus esculentus)* yields both a fiber and an edible fruit. This fruit, also called gumbo, is probably of African origin and is used in the French cookery of Louisiana. It is used in stews, soups and gravies, either dried or fresh.

Olive *(Olea europaea)* is an important food plant. The fruit is eaten and the oil extracted. Olive oil is an indispensable part of Italian and Greek cooking. "The olive is significant of security and peace, because it was with the olive-branch that the dove returned to the ark" (Skinner, *Myths & Legends,* p. 202, see Bibliography).

The Olive tree is the goddess Minerva's tree, she is the goddess of handicrafts. The Olive was cultivated in ancient Egypt and thus has been in continuous use as a food plant for over four thousand years.

Onions, Leeks and Shallots *(Allium spp.)* have been found in all ancient cultures, and then as now extensively used in cooking. What good soup stock or stew could be made without an Onion? They are used cosmetically for acne and skin disease, and medicinally for their expectorant, diuretic, and antiseptic qualities. Among other things, Onions, Leeks and Shallots have been found to balance blood pressure and to cleanse the body from "the inside to the outside." They contain sulphur, vitamins, mineral salts and protein.

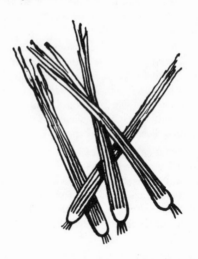

Recently I went to Maui for a hike across the Haleakala crater and stopped in Lahaina on my way home for a case of the famous Maui potato chips and a twenty-five-pound bag of the equally famous Maui Onions. Those Onions and I have had a marvelous time this last month getting to know one another. I have eaten Onions in every conceivable way: baked, boiled, stuffed, souped, stewed, saladed, raw with salt, and with all the traditional herbs and spices. At this point my favorite Onion recipe is simply to slice one thickly, put the slices into a heavy iron skillet with a teaspoon of mixed oils, toss in a few sliced Mushrooms, add a few cloves of crushed Garlic, sprinkle some Lovage or Tarragon, over the top and sauté over a low flame until the Onion is tender. This is a delicious and simple way to eat an Onion; it is a good recipe for a diet, as there are only about 150 calories in this dish and with a few Lettuce leaves, it is enough to make a satisfying lunch. If you have the opportunity, do try Maui Onions as they are sweeter and more delicate than any other Onion I have ever met.

The Onion is a magical plant and symbolized the universe to the Egyptians, "since in their cosmogony the various spheres of hell, earth, and heaven were concentric,"* like the layers of the Onion.

Oranges, Orange Peel, Orange Flowers *(Citrus sinensis)* and other Citrus fruits are much used in cookery (see also Lemon and Citron). The Orange flowers symbolize chastity, hence their use in bridal bouquets. Orange flowers and Orange flower water are used in fine cookery where the scent may also act as an aphrodisiac. The flowers can be infused in butter to spread on sweet breads, or in ice cream. Add the flower water to coffee for a delicious change in your morning brew. Cocktails, ices, sugars and liqueurs can be enhanced with the addition of the flower water or essential oil. The flower water is thought to be a mild soporific and can be taken by the teaspoonful at night before bedtime. Orange peel is candied and added to desserts, or eaten with the Orange for its bioflavonoid content. Orange juice syrup is delicious over crêpes and waffles.

Orchids *(Orchis spp.)* produce few plants that are used in cookery. Salep, sometimes used in love potions, was once an important food. Orchid flowers are used to dress up rum drinks; *Vanilla planifolia* yields the seed pod Vanilla which is used in pastries, drinks, sweets, and perfumery.

Pansies *(Viola tricolor)*, also called Heartsease because it was used as a heart tonic, is a medicinal herb that contains salicylic acid, tannin, glucosides, salts, alkaloids and vitamins. It can be chopped and used in salads, and the flowers in syrups, salads or wine. It is used as a specific for the skin.

Papaya *(Carica Papaya)* is a delicious fruit that can only really be enjoyed picked fresh from the tree. The best Papaya I ever tasted was shared with a new friend in Haleakala crater after a long hike (we also had a Mango, an Avocado and some Maui potato chips). They have received much attention recently because of their ability to clean old dirty wounds simply by applying fresh slices directly to the skin. They are also excellent digestives and can be eaten raw or juiced.

Paprika (see Capsicum).

Parsley *(Petroselinum crispum)* is one of the most popular seasoning herbs and foods and an extremely rich source of various minerals and vitamins, including Vitamins C and A. It is biennial, occasionally difficult to grow, and is used rather freely in all foods including sauces, soups, fish, eggs, meats, breads, and herbal mixtures. It is an important part of any reducing diet as it is a diuretic. An old remedy for cancer and

*(Skinner, *Myths & Legends*, p. 205).

skin growths is an ointment made of Violets, Parsley, Red Clover and Pansies. The Parsley was dedicated to Persephone, the queen of Hades and important in the funeral rites of the ancient Greeks. It is reputed to have grown from the blood of Archemorus, the Greek hero who is the forerunner of death.

▲**Passionflower** *(Passiflora incarnata)* is a plant whose flower is used in soups and syrups, and whose fruit *(P. edulis)* is delicately delicious and more often made into juice than eaten raw.

Peach and Peach Blossoms *(Prunus Persica)*. The Peach is a delicious fruit best eaten out of hand, but also used in syrups and liqueurs. The blossoms can be added to salads or made into syrups, conserves, teas and butters. All parts of the plant have a sedative action.

Pelargoniums (see Geranium).

▲**Pennyroyal** *(Mentha Pulegium)* has the power to drive away fleas, and was used by sailors to purify water. It is rarely used in cookery, although the infusion can cure obstructed menstruation.

Pepper *(Piper nigrum)*. Whereas Chile is a stimulant to the digestive tract, Pepper is an irritant. But it is ubiquitous in our seasoning of foods and has been used continuously since the time of Hippocrates (450 B.C.). The Pepper is the dried unripe fruit of the vine and was so valuable at one time that one's rent was demanded in Peppercorns.

Pine of all types can be used in cookery. Their needles have a woodsy scent and taste, contain much Vitamin C, and can be used to flavor game such as venison, and game birds such as quail or grouse. Pines also furnish edible seeds that are very high in proteins (such as Pinon nut), and these can be eaten raw or used in various sauces.

▲**Plantain** *(Plantago major)* contains an enormous amount of minerals and probably Vitamins A, C and K. It has somewhat of a tough taste, but the young leaves can be chopped and added to salads, used as a potherb, or in soups and stews. The green seeds are crunchy and nutritious and can be eaten raw, added to salads, various cereals and breads. Plantain was called White Man's footsteps for wherever white men went, the Plantain was sure to follow. It also symbolizes the path of Christ as he walked among the people. This plant is called Waybread by the Saxons who valued it highly, and in the old herbal, *Lacnunga,* it is mentioned as one of their nine sacred herbs.

Plantain *(Musa paradisiaca)*. See Banana.

▲**Pomegranate** *(Punica Granatum)* has been used since ancient Egyptian days (1500 BC), as both a medicine and a food. It symbolizes fecundity because of its many seeds.

Poppy *(Papaver somniferum)* seeds are sprinkled on rolls and breads, and used in pastry, cakes, and herbal mixtures such as Curry blends. Poppy seeds taste good on vegetables, rice, noodles, and on some kinds of light fish.

Potato *(Solanum tuberosum)* is a Peruvian import and was introduced into Europe in the late 1500's. They are a delicious food best eaten baked with a bit of butter and herb salt, but of course can be added to stews, salads, soups and casseroles. The raw juice contains potassium and this is useful in diets or applied externally for sores, black eyes or bruises.

▲Primrose (see Cowslips).

Psyllium Seeds *(Plantago Psyllium)* contain a mucilage that is sometimes used in cooking, but more often used medicinally for treating intestinal troubles.

Pumpkin *(Cucurbita Pepo).* The ancient civilizations of Central and South America made much use of the Beans, Corn, Pumpkins and Squashes. The Pumpkin is a fruit that stores well and can be used as a shell for other foods to be baked in. All parts of the plant are edible; the flowers are delicious fried as fritters, the seeds are an important part of Mexican cuisine, and the fruit itself can be baked, boiled, fried or roasted. Pumpkin seeds contain rather large amounts of protein and oil, and are a necessary addition to the diet. They will help keep the prostate gland healthy (see also Melons).

Purslane *(Portulaca sativa)* is 92% water, and contains some calcium, phosphorus, Vitamin A, iron, and other essential elements. It is among the most common of weeds and is found everywhere. Think of all the nutrition going to waste because you have not learned to identify the common purslane. It is usually used fresh as a potherb or added sparingly to salads. In ancient times purslane was thought to be an anti-magic herb, and was strewn generously around the room and the bed to protect the sleeper from evil spirits. Medicinally, purslane is a useful tonic for the blood.

Pyracantha produces edible berries that make good jelly or sauce.

▲Quince (various species of *Pyrus, Cydonia*) produces a delicious edible fruit sacred to Venus and thought to be the "golden Apple" of Virgil. Pliny goes into much detail concerning the medicinal value of the quince. The seed is mucilaginous and is often used in cosmetic preparation.

Radish *(Raphanus sativus)* is said by M. Grieve to be an effective food remedy for stone and gravel in the body.

Red Root (see *Lachantes tinctoria*).

Rhubarb *(Rheum rhaponticum)* is thought to be native to Asia Minor and was used medicinally as early as 2700 B.C. in China. The leaf is mildly poisonous, but the stems or petioles can be stewed and used in sauces and pies. They have a mild laxative (cleansing) action with an after-astringency that is useful in diarrhea. The flowers are also edible and can be fried as fritters.

Rice *(Oryza sativa)* is one of the three great cereal plants of the world. Rice has been grown and used since 3000 B.C. in China, and was introduced into Egypt about 700 A.D. by Arab traders. Rice is the only one of these important cereals that is eaten directly as harvested (corn is mostly fed to animals and man eats the meat, and wheat is milled to flour and then baked).

Rooibosch *(Aspalathus linearis)* tea is caffeine free and has a low tannin content, and so makes an ideal alternative to tea and coffee, and therefore it cannot cause the digestive disturbances produced by these two important beverages. It contains Vitamin C, protein and minerals such as iron, manganese, calcium, magnesium, and potassium. The tea has been used by people who have allergies, such as babies suffering from milk allergies. It is drunk as a tea, used in marinades, or in baking (see "Rooibosch Tea" by Bruce Ginsberg, *The Herbal Review,* Vol. 2, No. 2, 1977).

Roselle (see Hibiscus).

Rosemary *(Rosmarinus officinalis)* is one of my five most important plants (Garlic, Comfrey, Rosemary, Rose, and Camomile), and I use it in every conceivable way, from medicine to cosmetics to cooking. My father grew Rosemary as a ground cover and kept me well supplied with this fantastic herb. The flowers can be eaten or put into salads, and the herb is used in everything from garnishes to desserts and jellies. Try a sprig of fresh Rosemary under meat, or with Garlic inside a roasting chicken. It has a heady scent of much value in sleep pillows, if you want to have a restful night of sleep and to wake up refreshed in the morning. Rosemary butter is delicious over most vegetables, especially Eggplant and Peas. If you substitute Rosemary tea for the water that you would ordinarily use when making Lemonade, you will have a delicious drink that is useful to improve the memory, as Rosemary is one of the herbs specifically good for the brain.

Roses are a group of herbaceous shrubs which are one of my five most important plants. All parts, the leaves, petals, essence, and hips, are used medicinally, cosmetically, environmentally, and in the kitchen. I have three cookbooks alone that were written about the Rose and the things that one can do with it. Try making Rosewater, Rose petal biscuits, Rose petal jelly or jam, Rose hip syrup, Rose petal candles, Rose custard, Rose honey, Rose petal or Rose hip punch, Rose soda, Rose tinted ice cubes, Rose petal eggs (see Chapter 7), Rose poached fish, Rose ham, Rose frosting; OR Rose cosmetics such as those listed in *The Herbal Body Book;* OR environmental things such as Rose potpourri, Rose deodorizer; OR Rose medicine such as Rose petal cough syrup. These are a few of the recipes that could incorporate Roses (see *The Art of Cooking With Roses* by Jean Gordon).

Rose Hips are the swollen receptacles containing the hairy fruit left after the blossom dies, and are a natural source of Vitamin C: the more northerly the clime, the higher the content of Vitamin C. This vitamin begins to be lost as soon as the hip is picked, and so the picking must be done quickly and carefully to preserve as much of the vitamin as possible. Pick the hips in the fall when they are thoroughly ripe (bright red) and slightly soft to the touch (but not old and wrinkled). Dry them whole or cut in half. You can put them on trays in front of a warm (250°F.) oven to speed up the drying. But remember, heat also destroys Vitamin C. As soon as the hips are dry, put them in paper bags and store in a cool, dry place. Long storage causes the deterioration of the fruit and results in the loss of vitamin, so please use up those hips within a year of picking. When you make recipes using Rose hips, use a minimum amount of heat for a minimum time to retain as much Vitamin C as possible.

Safflower *(Carthamus tinctorius)* is a thistle-like plant, originally used for its red and yellow coloring matter. This color mixed with talc was called "rouge," and when mixed with Saffron, adulterates it. It certainly reduces the quality, color and flavor of Saffron (so only buy Saffron whole and *not* powdered). In comparatively recent times, Safflower has been cultivated for its unsaturated seed oil that is high in linoleic components, and which is used in margarines, mayonnaise, and other types of food products.

Saffron *(Crocus sativus)* is the stigmas of a crocus that flowers in the fall. Saffron is possibly the oldest known perfume and dye plant. Spain produces most of the world's Saffron, but 4000 acres are devoted to it in Kashmir, India. Saffron is an indispensable part of bouillabaisse, paella, and a number of other Spanish dishes. It can be used with rice, veal, fish, chicken, or cakes. It takes over 3000 blossoms to make 1 ounce of Saffron spice.

Sage *(Salvia officinalis,* white Sage, common Sage, red Sage; *S. mellifera,* black Sage). As Skinner p. 263 so adeptly puts it, "In the middle ages, when plants were much more remarkable than now, the common Sage prolonged life, heightened spirits, kept off toads, enabled girls to see their future husbands, mitigated sorrow, and averted chills." Sage is an old favorite in the kitchen and is used to counteract the rich greasiness of fatty meats. It is used in the stuffings of goose, duck, and pork, is cooked with poultry, rabbit, eggs, cheeses, Beans, Onions, and Tomatoes, and is added to salads, condiments or herbal tea blends. It is an herb that dries you up (checks excessive discharge from any part of the body); if you have a runny nose, loose bowels, too much urine, sweat too much, or have too much breast milk, then add Sage to your diet.

St.-John's-Wort *(Hypericum perforatum)* is an aromatic, astringent herb used as a tea before bedtime by bed-wetters. The red juice is useful in salves and is thought to represent the blood of John the Baptist. The flowers can be used in salads while the whole herb is occasionally used in liqueurs.

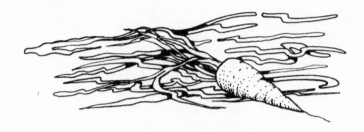

Salsify *(Tragopogon porrifolius)* is called the vegetable oyster because its flavor is reminiscent of the oyster. It is esteemed as a survival food, and can be steamed with lemon and butter, or grated and formed into patties.

Samphire *(Crithmum maritimum,* the umbel; *Salicornia herbacea* the goosefoot*)* are diuretic plants cultivated for their culinary uses as a potherb, pickle, or salad ingredient. They have been in use hundreds of years.

Santolina Chamaecyparissus, or Lavender cotton, is used in stocks, soups and stews, especially where the meat is greasy; it can also be used with vegetables such as Zucchini.

▲**Sassafras** *(Sassafras officinale)* is a native inhabitant of the United States, the bark being used as a vascular dilator, and the leaves an important ingredient in sauces, soups, gumbo, and condiments. In the 1800s, Saloop, a kind of tea made with Sassafras was a common drink in England.

Savory *(Satureja hortensis,* summer Savory; *S. montana, winter Savory).* Summer Savory is an annual, while Winter Savory is a perennial, and they are a traditional accompaniment to Beans. They are good chopped into salads, rubbed on bee stings to relieve swelling and pain, used in Onion, Pea or Lentil soup, baked fish or roasted pork, added to herb vinegar and meat loaf, and served on Cauliflower or Beets.

Scurvy Grass *(Cochlearia officinalis)* is an herb of the order Cruciferae. It contains Vitamin C and was formerly carried on sea voyages to be eaten as a preventative of scurvy.

Sea Vegetables or Seaweeds (see also Kelp) are an important part of the diet of peoples living near the sea. Sea plants contain in greater or lesser degree all the vitamins and minerals needed in the diet. Some sea plants contain substances that combine with toxic elements in the body, enabling these elements to be harmlessly excreted. It is a good habit to eat some form of Sea vegetable every day. Sea plants, usually dried, can be found in any grocery specializing in Oriental food products, and recipes for them can be found in Japanese cookbooks. Many communities are now giving plant identification classes that also include edible Sea plants. Agar-agar, or kanten, which is made from a red algae, is used as a gelling agent for aspic, dessert, salads or soup (this is important for vegetarians who wish to find a substitute for animal gelatins).

Sesame *(Sesamum indicum),* also called Benne or Ben, is a staple food in several countries. It has been grown in Asia since ancient times. Both the seed and the oil are used. The seed when ground is called tahini and used in various regional cuisines, notably Greek and Turkish. Tahini, when mixed with cooked ground Garbanzo Beans, makes a delicious complete protein that can be eaten as a dessert or as a dip, depending on the seasonings used (see Chapter 14). The toasted seeds are a tasty addition when used on vegetables, salads, potatoes or meats, and when mixed with sea salt can decrease the amount of salt used (2 parts toasted seeds to 1 part salt, ground together in a seed mill). Sesame oil is a semi-drying oil that can be used in cooking or on salads.

Skirret *(Sium Sisarum)* is a plant grown for its tuberous root, eaten rather like Salsify. It is a perennial grown as an annual to produce the best tasting roots.

Sorghum *(Sorghum vulgare)* or Broomcorn, is widely cultivated as a grain, sweetener (Sorghum syrup), and forage crop. It has a great resistance to drought, but becomes rancid rather easily after milling, and so is not extensively grown here.

Sorrel *(Rumex scutatus,* French Sorrel; *R. Acetosa,* wild or garden Sorrel) is slightly astringent, and contains much Vitamin C and oxalic acid. This plant is used as a slightly acid-tasting potherb, and in the famous French Sorrel soup. Since it contains oxalic acid, which combines with calcium to form an insoluble salt, it should not be mixed or eaten with milk. It also should not be cooked in iron pans as it will pick up the metallic taste. It can be added to greasy foods such as pork, scrambled with eggs, chopped and added to salads, wrapped around fish and baked, cooked with Lentils, and, in general, used in many sauces and soups.

Southernwood *(Artemisia Abrotanum),* also called Old Man or Lad's Love because it is said to grow hair on the face of a young man or on the bald head of an old man, is quite aromatic and can be added sparingly to salads. In Italy it is added to cakes.

Sow Thistle *(Sonchus oleraceus)* is a common backyard weed that was at one time added with other plants in salads and soups.

Spinach *(Spinacia oleracea)* is another plant that is a member of the goosefoot family which seems to have so many edible members. The comic strip character Popeye ate Spinach for its iron content, but nettles are better for supplying iron. New Zealand Spinach *(Tetragonia expansar)* is an edible Spinach which is not a member of the goosefoot family of plants.

Star Anise (see Anise).

Stonecrops *(Sedum spp.)* are natural seasonings because of their peppery taste.

Sunflowers *(Helianthus annuus)* are tall striking annuals, sometimes growing ten feet in a season. An "obvious symbol of the globe of light," they were much esteemed by the sun-worshipping Incas of Peru. Their sun priestesses wore gold crowns that were copies of the sunflower "to the great joy of the Spaniards, who immediately possessed themselves of these shocking evidences of the unauthorized religion, and put the priestesses to the sword." (Skinner, *Myths and Legends,* p. 273).

Sunflower seeds are roasted and eaten with a great cracking sound, as every schoolteacher knows, and the raw or roasted seeds are of great benefit to the male reproductive organs. Sunflower oil is delicious and can be used to fry potato chips and make a salad dressing.

Sweet Cicely *(Myrrhis odorata)* is used as a tonic tea for a young girl's first menstrual cycles. It is also a "sweet" plant found useful by diabetics, used in soups and stews, fresh in salads, for diets and fasting, for stewing fruits, and as a flavoring for cakes.

Tansy *(Tanacetum vulgare)* has a very bitter taste, is used for menstrual difficulties, and formerly was much used in cookery, especially during Lent.

Tapioca (see Manioc).

Tarragon *(Artemisia Dracunculus).* There are two types of tarragon, the Russian variety and the French. The French tarragon is the only one acceptable in French cuisine. Called the king of the culinary herbs, it has a tart, somewhat sweet licorice taste, and is essential in Béarnaise or Hollandaise sauce. Tarragon is often combined with chervil, and used in many foods, from condiments, eggs and fruits, to meats and sauces.

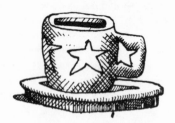

▲ **Tea** *(Camellia (Thea) sinensis),* also called *cha,* is the dried leaf tip of this plant native to China and India. Tea trading was the backbone of the East India Trading Company, and Tea drinking gradually replaced the Coffee of the New World as the major beverage in England and her colonies. To offset the high tannin content of Tea, it is good to drink it with milk. Tea leaves are sometimes eaten with butter and salt.

Thistles of many kinds are eaten and enjoyed. The Artichoke is one Thistle we eat for its tasty flower, while the Milk Thistle is used as a potherb as well as a galactogue. The common Sow Thistle is alien to the United States and was originally imported from Europe, can be used as a potherb, or the young leaves added to salads.

Thyme *(Thymus vulgaris,* common thyme; *T. citriodorus,* Lemon Thyme; *T. Herba-Barona,* Caraway Thyme) is a little plant with a big flavor. It was once used to cover the scent of rotting meat and as a strewing herb, and has great medicinal value. There is an incredible range in the flavors and scents of Thymes: from Nutmeg, Caraway, Mint, Pine, and Pepper to Lemon, Citronella, Camphor, and many more. In our home, we regularly use the common, the Lemon, and the Caraway Thyme. Thyme honey is particularly desirable. Thymes are important ingredients in herb vinegar, on vegetables such as Beans, Onions and Tomatoes, in Bouquet Garni, to season game birds, in egg and cheese dishes, in herb butters and sauces, in stuffings and salads, and in vegetable and meat soups. Lemon Thyme goes well with fish, while Caraway Thyme is good in herb butters and breads. Thyme is an antiseptic herb and is very good in aiding digestion. It has been recommended to be used in beer soup to cure shyness, and likes to live next to Lavender. Because Thyme is an antiseptic herb, it can be used in facial steam mixtures to cleanse the skin; try mixing Thyme with Camomile to reduce puffiness, with Licorice to open the pores for cleansing, and with Comfrey for cellular regeneration.

▲**Tonka Bean** *(Dipteryx odorata)* has been used as a substitute for vanilla. Its delicious odor is due to the presence of coumarin, an anti-coagulant which also occurs in such plants as Woodruff, Melilot and some Clovers. The plant has somewhat of a narcotic effect when taken immoderately; once, when I used it in waffles, I became rather dizzy and disoriented. The waffles, however, were delicious.

▲**Tragacanth** *(Astragalus gummifer)* is a gum used in making lozenges, cough drops, cosmetics, liqueurs, and dental creams.

▲**Tuberose** *(Polianthes tuberosa)* is a wonderfully fragrant plant. The flowers continue to exhale their perfume long after being picked, and they can be added to wines, teas, or salads, and made into candy or flower water. They act to enhance all the senses and the scent is an aphrodisiac. In the language of flowers, the Tuberose symbolizes dangerous pleasures.

Tulip *(Tulipa spp.).* The pistils of Tulips can be removed and the Tulip stuffed with chicken or tuna salad. Many plants can be used as natural bowls and plates.

Tupelo *(Nyssa spp.)* is a tree with small greenish flowers and bluish or purple fruit. It is native to the southeastern United States and is also called the Cotton Gum tree. The honey is delicious and is useful to diabetics because it has a different type of sugar with a sugar content lower than in other types of honey.

Turmeric *(Curcuma longa)* belongs to the same family as the Ginger, and like Ginger, the spice Turmeric comes from the underground rhizome. Turmeric is sweet and quite fragrant, is bright yellow, and is used both as a culinary plant and a dye plant. Turmeric is used in Curry powder mixtures, sprinkled on eggs, and gives color and flavor to mayonnaise, salad dressings, drinks, and liqueurs.

▲**Vanilla** *(Vanilla planifolia)* is the picked and fermented fruit of the vanilla, an orchid vine. It is certainly a unique flavoring agent with a taste best described as Vanilla-like. The Aztecs used Vanilla with chocolate drinks. We use Vanilla in drinks, desserts, foods, tobacco, perfumery and liqueurs. In other times, Vanilla was thought to be medicinal, and can be used as an aid for the digestion, as well as being an aphrodisiac. Tonka beans have on occasion been substituted for the Vanilla in recipes.

Verbena, Lemon (see Lemon Verbena).

Vernal Grass *(Anthoxanthum odoratum)* smells somewhat like new-mown hay or Sweet Melilot. A tincture of Vernal Grass snuffed in the nose is thought to give relief from hay fever and asthma. The taste is good and it can be used in teas, mixed with other herbs, or used to flavour liqueurs.

Vine (see Grape).

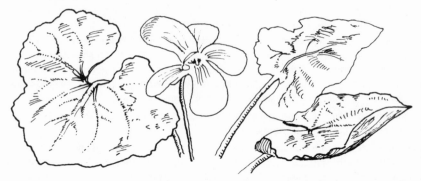

Violet *(Viola odorata)* has many uses in cookery. They have a delicious fragrance, but a slightly bitter taste. Violet leaves contain glucosides, and the entire plant is rather rich in Vitamin C and salicin. Tea made from this plant has been used as a specific for throat cancer, while the flower syrup has been used as a cough remedy, laxative, and to soothe nerves. Inhaling the scent of Violets is good to relax the mind and relieve stress. Violets have been candied, used in salads, mixed with Fennel and Savory for soup, cooked with salmon to give it a unique flavor, and made into jellies, teas, candies and conserves. The flowers also give a lovely tint and taste when infused in vinegar for salad dressings. This plant belongs to Venus and it has been much used in cosmetics.

Wallflower *(Cheiranthus Cheiri)* flowers can be used in salads, while the entire plant is a specific for the muscles and sinews.

Walnut *(Juglans nigra)* contains protein, is much used in foods, garnishes and desserts, or is simply eaten by hand. The bark and leaves are generally used medicinally for treating skin problems. In the Doctrine of Signatures, the Walnut resembles the brain and its many coverings, and is thus used for diseases of the head; the Walnut oil, for instance, has a reputation for growing hair on the baldest pate.

Watercress *(Nasturtium officinale)* is a delicious addition to salads and soups. It is "also called scurvy grass. This plant grows in slow moving streams. It is very high in Vitamins C and E, has a higher percentage of organic minerals than Spinach, and has no oxalic acid. It contains manganese and is used as a blood builder, to nourish the pituitary glands, is stimulating to the digestion, can clear the skin of pimples and sores, and is eaten to dissolve kidney stones."* It is also of much value in reducing diets.

Wisteria *(Wisteria sinensis)* is a hardy climbing plant from China where it is used as a diuretic. Its seeds are thought to preserve wine from spoiling, and if the wine is spoiled will restore it. We can use Wisteria flowers in salads, fritters, preserves or wine. In the Language of Flowers it means, "I cling to thee."

Woodruff *(Asperula odorata)* is the herb used in German new wines to give it good flavor, called May wine. The fragrance of this lovely little plant develops as it dries and is due to an anti-coagulant substance called coumarin. It is usually collected in woods and can be used in drinks, teas, cakes, sauces, and when cooking chicken.

▲**Wormwood** *(Artemisia absinthium)* was once used to flavor a drink called absinthe, but it is toxic when used over a long period of time, and thought to derange the mind. The plant is occasionally used in cookery to make tea and brew beer, but it has an extremely bitter taste and is now mostly used for its medicinal qualities.

Yerba Buena *(Satureja Douglasii)* is a Mint with a strong aromatic fragrance used in South American cookery, especially in Cuban food. It goes well in meat sauces and can be used in teas.

Yerba Maté *(Ilex paraguariensis)* is the herb tea drunk daily by more than 30 million South Americans. It contains much caffeine and tannin, and when taken in quantity acts as a diuretic, (to pee more), a diaphoretic, (to sweat more), and a tonic. It is specially made in a gourd and sucked out with a tube, rather than drunk out of a cup. Maté goes well with other herbs and is useful as a substitute for coffee.

▲**Yohimbe** *(Pausinystalia yohimbe)* is usually thought of as a tea herb used as an aphrodisiac, but one of my former students who used it frequently said that it tasted terrible, and so he has experimented with other ways to ingest Yohimbe. He suggests that you grind it in a blender, mix it with other marinade ingredients, and marinate your meat in this mixture before you roast or barbeque. He said that it "goes right through the meat," rendering it tender.

*Jeanne Rose, *Herbs & Things*, p. 113.

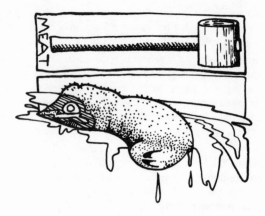

Some of the books referred to for Latin binomials include:

Hortus Third. Staff of the L. H. Bailey Hortorium, Cornell University. New York: Macmillan Co., 1976.
Schery, Robert W. *Plants for Man.* Second edition. New Jersey: Prentice-Hall, 1972.
Grieve, Mrs. M. A Modern Herbal. New York: Hafner Publishing Co., 1931 and 1971.

Chapter 4

Special Tables and Lists

WEIGHTS AND MEASURES

Soon we shall finally be caught up with the rest of the world by going metric in this country—so we ought to learn how to measure in this system. It is not hard to learn metrics; it just requires that we change our thinking habits and start USING the system.

First, we have to learn a few basic words.

WEIGHT is measured in GRAMS (pounds and ounces)

VOLUME is measured in LITERS (cups, fluid ounces, or quarts)

LENGTH is measured in METERS (feet or inches)

Second, we have to go back to some Latin roots that we might have been introduced to in high school to learn a few of the important prefixes of the metric system.

MILLI means 1/1000 or one-thousandth

CENTI means 1/100 or one-hundredth

KILO means 1000 times one or one thousand times

Now all we have to do is put the prefix with the base word and we have a measure, such as a milligram is 1/1000 of a gram, and a kilogram is 1000 grams.

Lastly, we have to remember that water will boil at the same degree of heat but the names of the degrees will change. Now we will use both the terms "celsius" (centigrade) and "Fahrenheit" to describe temperature, p.e. water boils at 100°C. or 212°F.

Scales For

Celsius	0°	20°	37°	100°	150°	200°
Fahrenheit	32°	68°	98.6° Body Temp	212°	318°	424°

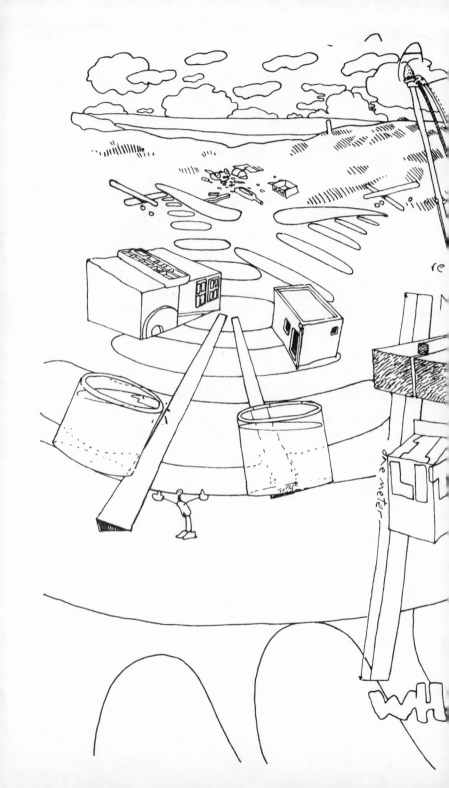

re

ane meter

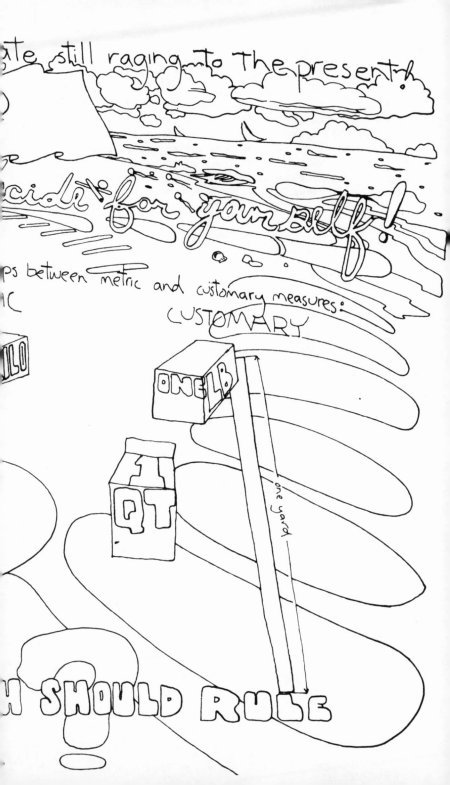

In this book most of the recipes will use measurements by the cup, ounce, teaspoon and tablespoon. But many of my recipes, because they have been handed down from mother or father to daughter, and because the ingredients have been changed around to suit the time of year or the contents of one's refrigerator, will use what I consider to be a more reliable system of measure. That is by the "handful" or "to taste" system. This is particularly good because the food can be seasoned to one's own taste rather than according to my taste, (which is bizarre, some might say).

Basic Measurements

1 t. = ⅓ T.	16 T. = 1 C.
3 t. = 1 T.	2 C. = 1 pt.
4 T. = ¼ C.	4 C. = 1 qt.
	4 qt. = 1 gallon

Abbreviations Used in This Book

°F.—degrees Fahrenheit	C.—cup
°C.—centigrade or celsius degrees	pt.—pint
t.—teaspoon(s)	qt.—quart
T.—tablespoon(s)	oz.—ounce(s)
fl. oz.—fluid ounce(s)	lb.—pound

TABLE 5

TABLE OF EQUIVALENTS

American Measure

Liquid			Solid IN GRAMS	
1 t.	1/6 fl. oz.	5 ml.	5 g.	
1 T. (3t.)	½ fl. oz.	15 ml.	15 g.	
1 C. (16T.)	8 fl. oz.	227 ml.	227 g.	
1 pt. (2C.)	16 fl. oz.	454 ml.	454 g.	1 lb.

Imperial Measure

1 pt.	20 fl. oz.		16 oz.	1 lb.
1 qt. (slightly less than 4C.)	2 pt.			
1 gal.	4 qt.			
1 lb.			16 oz.	

Metric Measure

1 oz.	30 g.
1 lb.	½ kg. or 500 g.
1 fl. oz.	30 ml.
1 pt.	½ liter, approximately

Other Measures

A list of apothecary measures and symbols is in *Herbs & Things* is suitable for translating some of the measuring systems used in old herbals, and in *The Herbal Body Book* you will find measurements useful in the creation of fine body care products.

CULINARY EQUIPMENT

If you are starting a kitchen from scratch, a situation I cannot even imagine, you will have to have a certain number of basic tools and cooking items. These tools are listed in alphabetical order, as that makes the most sense to me, but you will most certainly find that a number of items you consider to be basic are missing. These items will probably be in the realm of pieces of equipment used in the making of sweets and pastries, as I feel these are totally unnecessary items in one's diet. I also have extremely strong feelings about grains, and the fact that we don't really need to eat them, or meat, which in this country seems to be overeaten and overused. If we would only eat about half of what we normally consume, and exercise twice as much, we would improve our health to a marvelous degree, and certainly would save an enormous amount of money from reduced grocery bills.

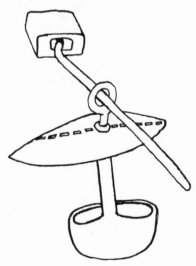

TABLE 6   **BASIC COOKING ITEMS**

basting or pastry brush
bean pot
blender or mixer
bottle opener
bowl—a copper bowl for adding air into egg
      whites for soufflés
bowls—a set of mixing bowls
bowl—a wooden salad bowl
bread pans
can opener
canisters or glass containers
coffee maker
colander
cookbooks—an assortment of good
                cookbooks
cookie sheets—for granola
corkscrew
cutting board
Dutch oven (cast-iron)
Dutch oven (enamel) or soup kettle
fondue maker
food mill
funnels—a couple of funnels
grater
herbs
knives—a set of knives, especially a paring
        knife and a chopping knife
ladle
measuring cups
measuring spoons
mortar and pestle
pan—a nice sautépan or wok
pasta pot or deep enamel pot with colander
    type insert
pie pan or quiche pan
pot holders
roasters—a set of roasters
rolling pin
rubber spatula

saucepans—2 enamel or glass saucepans with
            lids or double boiler
scales
seed grinder
skillet—large cast-iron skillet
skillet—a small cast-iron skillet
soup ladle
soup tureen
spatula
squeezer—lemon or orange squeezer
strainers—some different sizes
straining cloths
tea set or pot
timer
tongs
vegetable parer
vegetable scrub brush
waffle iron
wire whisk
wooden spoons

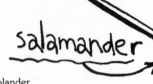

salamander

HERBS FOR THE SENSE OF TASTE

"Good food and good cooking are rapidly disappearing, and the sense of taste is dependent on both these things and has to be cultivated to reach the fullest enjoyment," so wrote Mrs. C. F. Leyel in *Cinquefoil* (p. 211, see Bibliography). "Taste is the sense by means of which we prove the sapidity and esculence of things" is the definition of taste given by Brillat-Savarin. There are specific herbs for the sense of taste and for the good health of the mouth, taste buds, and tongue, just as there are specific herbs for all the other senses. There are four basic taste sensations: sweet, bitter, sour, and salty. And there are specific herbs that represent these taste sensations as well as specific herbs that balance them if they are overly strong in any one direction.

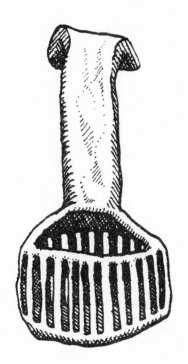

TABLE 7

SENSATION	HERB	HERB TO BALANCE
Sweet	Licorice	Sabadilla
Bitter	Golden Seal	Dandelion
Sour	Lemon Peel	Carnations & Pinks
Salty	Dulse	Cyclamen

To improve your sense of taste, relax a bit and eat slowly, and leisurely enjoy each bite. If you do not have enough time to do this, then it is far better to skip the meal rather than eat in a hurried manner. Eat half as much, but make sure that what you eat is of the highest quality. You will probably save money, lose weight from eating less, and enjoy life more. Meanwhile, your sense of taste will definitely improve.

Common Name	Scientific Name	Function
Anemone	*(Anemone pulsatilla)*	For loss of smell and for extremely emotional people given to extremes of pleasure and misery
▲Arum (Cuckoo-pint)	*(Arum triphyllum)*	For sore mouth
Bird's Foot	*(Lotus corniculatus)*	To promote healthy mouth and cure spongy gums
Camomile	*(Camomilla matricaria)*	For hypersensitivity to ranges in smell and taste
Carnation	*(Dianthus carophyllus)*	To enliven all the senses and to cure an overly sour taste
Carob	*(Ceratonia siliqua)*	To clear the voice and to promote a healthy taste
Cheddar Pinks *(simple carnation)*	*(D. deltoides)*	To enliven all the senses and to correct any disorder of the head area
▲Christmas Rose	*(Helleborus niger)*	Enhances the sense of taste
▲Cinquefoil	*(Potentilla reptans)*	Love-divining herb used to promote healthy gum tissue
Dandelion	*(Taraxacum officinale)*	For a geographic tongue, loss of appetite, and to counteract bitter taste
Echinacea	*(E. angustifolia)*	To relieve dry, swollen or sore tongue; to cure mouth ulcers, cold sores or mouth herpes
Geranium	*(Geranium maculatum G. robertianum)*	For a continuous dry mouth or inflamed tongue
▲Ground Pine *(Yellow Bugle)*	*(Ajuga chamarpitys)*	Used as a mouth wash
Herb Patience	*(Rumex alpinus)*	For a perverted taste
Horse Chestnut	*(Aesculus hippocastanum)*	For a coated tongue or to remove a metallic taste in the mouth
▲Ipecac	*(Cephaelis ipecacuana)*	An amoebicide; to improve salivary secretion and to affect the sense of smell and taste
Jack Fruit	*(Artocarpus integrifolia)*	To promote a healthy state of the mouth
▲Lily of the Valley	*(Convallaria majalis)*	Flowers and leaves used to remove a coppery taste from the mouth and to heal a sore and scalded feeling on the tongue

Common Name	Scientific Name	Function
▲ Marsh Crowfoot	*(Ranunculus seleratus)*	A homeopathic tincture used for a geographic tongue and to relieve burning and hardness of the tongue
Mulberry	*(Morus alba), (M. nigra)*	For all problems relating to mouth and throat
Myrtle	*(Myrtus communis)*	For all mucous membranes, particularly for a furred tongue, bad taste in the mouth, and tender bleeding gums
Privet	*(Ligustrum vulgare)*	For spongy and bleeding gums
Rock Rose	*(Cistus canadensis)*	For swollen gums or a tongue that can only be extended with pain; for pyorrhea or a sore mouth.
Snapdragon	*(Antirrhinum orontium)*	Used specifically for the tongue; to cure a dry mouth or rough tongue; (used for liver derangement)
Stocks	*(Matthiola incarna)*	A cordial plant that appeals to all the senses and excellent in salads
Strawberries, Wild	*(Fragaria vesca)*	The juice dissolves tartar and promotes a healthy mouth
Sweet William	*(Dianthus barbatus)*	To enliven the senses and to correct any disorder in the head area
Tomato	*(Lycopersicum esculentum)*	To cure an ulcerated mouth
▲ Tormentilla	*(Potentilla tormentilla)*	An astringent used to heal mouth ulcers
Wintersweet	*(Chimonanthus fragrans)*	Specifically works on the salivary glands to increase or decrease their flow

For a more detailed account of the various herbs for the sense of taste see *Cinquefoil* by Mrs. C. F. Leyel.

Chapter 5

How to Collect, Use, and Store
Plants for Culinary Use

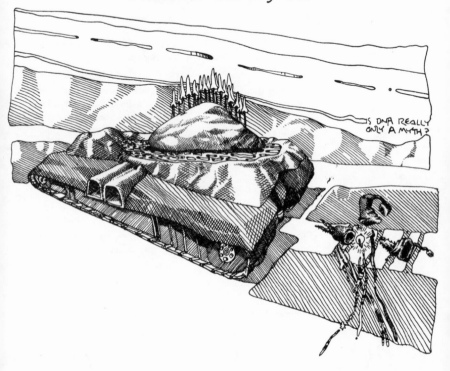

IS DNA REALLY ONLY A MYTH?

As I sat down to write this chapter it occurred to me that in my previous works, *Herbs & Things* and the *Herbal Body Book,* I had already written my ideas on the subject of gathering and collecting plants. It seemed a propitious time to get another's view on the growth and handling of herbal materials. The bio-dynamic method of growth and care of plants is one that I have always admired and so I contacted Heinz Grotzke of Meadowbrook Herb Garden, Wyoming, Rhode Island 02898, who uses this method to grow his fantastic herbs. He graciously gave me his permission to paraphrase his pamphlet, "Growing Quality Herbs." If you wish to receive it, or his regular catalog of fantastic herbs and cosmetics, simply send 50¢.

"The interest in herbs has continually increased over the past few years, and so has the number of people who wish to study their history and usefulness. In our own dealings with herbs and contacts with people we have accumulated sufficient evidence to underwrite this statement. Almost daily, inquiries reach us from individuals and organizations about herbs and their sources, each time challenging our knowledge of herbs anew. Sometimes it is surprising to hear what motives are given to explain the curiosity in herbs, though more often it is fascinating to listen to the expectations that herbs are to fulfill.

We, as practical commercial herb growers, try to accomplish one simple and yet demanding task above all others: To produce herb products of the highest quality obtainable. In reaching this goal, experience has taught us that this is possible by making use of the bio-dynamic agricultural methods. The quality we mean is a totality comprised of bio-dynamic fertilization and cleanliness in growing, purity and know-how in processing, and appearance, fragrance and excellence in packaging.

In a brief fashion let us acquaint you with our herbal involvement step by step, so that it may become clear why we do what we do, and to show you how to do it for yourselves so that you can grow, become familiar with and use herbs in your own daily lives.

GROWING

Growing plants begins with soil and its treatment. Propagate plants from seeds or cuttings. It is best to use composted manure as fertilizer and herbal and bio-dynamic sprays as regulators. Chopped hay can be used as a mulch to cover the soil (for cleanliness) and as additional food for soil life, especially for the earthworms. Earthworms are extremely important to plant life as they keep the surface of the earth renewed and convert any waste matter into top soil. Companion planting is also important and should be practiced whenever possible.* Ideal for raising flavorful herbs is a sandy loam type of soil. Geographic location and climate are equally important for quality and quantity of growth.

HARVESTING

The right time of harvest and the way harvesting itself is done determines to a great extent the quality of the final product. The herb to be harvested should be young enough to still display a full green color and yet old enough to have fully developed its essential oils and be in the first stage of flowering. The right moment, of course, varies

---

*Use *Companion Plant* by Philbrick and Gregg.

with each plant species. Cut the herbs by hand, high enough above ground to allow new shoots to develop for a second growth. Yellow leaves, leaves soiled by bird droppings or used by insects to pupate or hibernate, spears of grass, weeds, these all should be removed by hand before the herbs are placed into a basket. Line up the stems of the herbs in the same direction. Only then can the herbs be chopped up to reach a uniform particle size.

DRYING

Harvesting is followed immediately by the preparation for drying; in fact, while harvesting is still in progress, some people simultaneously spread the harvested and chopped herbs on screens to be drying while the harvesting still goes on. The herbs on the screens should also be checked again for any impurities. The immediate drying is ideal because herbs like Marjoram tend to heat up while in the baskets rather quickly, and should this happen, they lose color and fragrance. The screens can be racked or laid about in a warm, dry and dark place. The best drying temperature is 100° F. The herbs should be left on the screens for as long as it takes the specific herb to become brittle and dry enough for either rubbing, immediate storage, or further processing.

RUBBING

All herb mixtures and herb seasonings should be rubbed, which is a process that separates the leaves from the stems by pressing the leaves with a circular hand motion through a fine screen. The stems stay on top of the screen and are discarded and composted, while the broken-up leaves are rubbed once again and then dedusted before being put into jars for labeling.

STORAGE

Since most of the herbs cannot be immediately bottled after harvesting, these have to be placed in storage. A storage room or place should be clean, dry, dark and cool so that the herbs will not break down during the time they are being stored. Paper bags, cardboard cartons, covered glass jars are all suitable storage containers.

At Meadowbrook Herb Garden, once the culinary herbs have dried on the screens in the drying house, they are rubbed right in the drying house and then loaded into barrels. The tea herbs, in contrast, are dumped from the screens into a movable bin and from there scooped into the storage barrels. All this is done inside the drying house, with heat on, and under optimum conditions of dryness and controlled humidity, in order to prevent the herbs from picking up moisture again. Humidity or moisture are the greatest enemies of quality herbs, especially if they are meant to keep their quality until the consumer begins to use them in the kitchen.

WARNING

Herbs which pick up moisture again, after drying, begin from that moment on to deteriorate. The most noticeable indication is the loss of green color, caused by the gradual decomposition of the chlorophyll. This initial deterioration phase is followed by a loss of the desired aroma, which is replaced in time by a musty or moldy smell, thus making the entire material useless for flavoring.

SOLUTION

Meadowbrook Herb Garden's solution to the problem of deterioration of herbal material is to allow only properly packaged herbs to leave the premises. My personal solution to keeping dried plants from deteriorating is to store them properly and to immediately get rid of any herbs that have begun to break down.

STORAGE INSECTS

Moisture and humidity are the greatest enemies of quality of plants in storage. Closely following in their ability to spoil an herb's quality are most certainly various types of insects some of which are called "flour beetles." These insects can become a grevious nuisance in storage. Often fumigation will seem to be the answer to an insect infestation, but in our minds fumigation should never even be considered but on the other hand should be condemned. Fumigation will, without doubt, kill an insect infestation in stored herbs, but will not remove the insect themselves from the stored materials. One should think in terms of creating conditions that prevent insects from infesting rather than thinking in terms of getting rid of the little beasts once they have appeared in your herbs.

Humidity again is a decisive factor. Only under humid conditions and in damp herb materials can insects develop, live, or breed. Aside from taking precautions to avoid such conditions herbs can be stored in insect-proof containers such as mason jars with canning lids. Storage areas should be dark and dry.

LIGHT

Another factor which must be discouraged if you are to retain quality of herbs in storage is light. That is light, all forms of light from sunlight to electric light. All light has a bleaching effect upon the green-leaved herbs, which in time would turn from green to light grey.

PACKAGING

The best container in which to package herbs according to Meadowbrook is a clear glass spice jar easily purchased at any one of a number of department stores or kitchen supply places. However, I must say that I favor amber glass jars or clear glass that has been covered with sticky shelf paper to exclude the light.

SUMMARY

In summary, let me say that in order to grow and have available herbs of superior quality for your kitchen, you ought to do the following:

1) Bio-dynamic/organic growing
2) Picking over the herb material by hand in field and drying
3) Gently chopping the herbs by hand
4) Careful low-temperature drying
5) Hand rubbing through screens to remove stems
6) Controlled storage conditions
7) Careful packaging

USING CULINARY PLANTS

Forget everything that you have ever heard about using herbs in cooking. Most books say the same thing. "Use a pinch, don't use a heavy hand, don't add so much herbal seasoning that you actually taste the herb, use herbs to hint at flavor" and other statements that show me the authors really don't like the taste of the herbal seasoning. To heck with "pinches" and "dashes of." Herbs *are* food and they are loaded with necessary vitamins and minerals, and they can often be eaten in rather generous quantities. I love the taste of Tarragon and often use a teaspoonful in a scrambled egg. I *want* to taste the Tarragon and use the egg as seasoning. In Mexican cooking I use lots of Cumin and Oregano—I am certainly not afraid of using a generous hand in seasoning my food. The only exception to this is in the use of salt which I use sparingly or not at all. So don't be afraid; using herbs is great fun.

But remember that there is a difference between using fresh and dried herbs. A pot of tea made with a lot of dried Mint is certainly not the same pot of tea as one made with a tea pot full of freshly picked Mint. Try both kinds and see what I mean. There *are* differences in the taste of fresh and dried herbs. Pasta con Pesto is made and can only be made with fresh Basil—dried Basil simply won't do. But try squirting a drop of Basil oil on a large handful of dried Basil. Tightly cover it and store for a time and then use it in Pesto sauce; you will be agreeably surprised. The flavors you can attain, by spraying the essential oil of a plant upon itself after it has dried, are very interesting. This is a technique that I often use when I want the taste of a fresh herb but simply do not have it available. In this case, though, you must use an extremely light hand when spraying the herbs. This technique is also exceedingly useful when making potpourris.

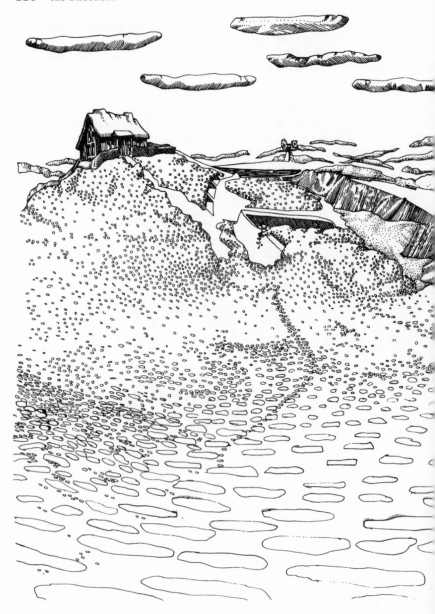

Chapter 6

Where and How to Purchase Those Exotic Ingredients and Delightful Cooking Goodies That You Have Longed for (Along with Some Other Items of Interest)

When I first became interested in producing herbal products, I found that the simple equipment required was very difficult to find. I had hunted in department stores, then changed my hunt to ethnic neighborhoods where I found much to my pleasure that all the equipment, interesting and odd cooking appliances, enamelware pots, and similar items were available. Today most department stores have well-stocked kitchen departments where the most exotic and esoteric items one could desire are available. However, even now you will usually find in ethnic neighborhoods odd little hardware stores, tucked away delicatessens, and small specialized groceries, and these are the places to go to get that wonderful sauce or that special type of pot that you have wanted. The prices will probably be less than in the big department stores and the search will be infinitely more rewarding.

Mail-order catalogs are also good places to go shopping. The prices often vary wildly from one catalog to another, but I have often found it simpler to go shopping sitting in my chair looking through a mail-order catalog than wandering around frantically from place to place looking for a simple tool that turned out to be necessary.

This list of stores is by no means complete* but it is a start. Do check the following sources for the items you desire.

Department store kitchen departments
Health food stores
Herbs in the telephone directory yellow pages
Herb stores
Neighborhood stores
Pharmacies, natural or homeopathic
Specialized stores for culinary goods and equipment

*List compiled in late 1976

ALABAMA

Priester's Pecans, 227 Old Fort Dr., Fort Deposit, Alabama 36032.
  Pecan and pecan products and fruitcakes. Mail-order catalog.

CALIFORNIA

Busy Bee Rabbitry, 315 B. St., Colma, California 94014.
  Here are all your rabbit needs, from live rabbits for pets to properly killed rabbits for food to good compost for your garden.

Fantasy Research Institute, P. O. Box 14305, San Francisco, California 94114.
  Sells various things by mail-order, including chlorella capsules, a pure natural source of quick energy.

Herb Products Company, 11012 Magnolia Blvd., No. Hollywood, California 91601. Mail-order catalog.

House of Almonds, P. O. Box 5125, Bakersfield, California 93308.
  Mail-order catalog.

Nature's Herb Company, 281 Ellis St., San Francisco, California 94102. Consistent, good quality in herbs and products. Mail-order catalog 50¢.

New Age Creations—Body Care & Books, 219 Carl St.,   San Francisco, California 94117.
  Pure, natural products, ingredients listed on the label, sometimes slow in shipping. Retail and wholesale. Mail-order catalog 50¢.

Saso Herb Gardens, 14625 Fruitvale Ave., Saratoga, California 95070.
  Wonderful organically grown herbs for sale, herb walks and talks. Louis and Virginia give frequent classes in all aspects of herbology. Write for dates.

Sunset House, 262 Sunset Bldg., Beverly Hills, California 90215. A few interesting cooking items among the other somewhat funky goodies. Mail-order catalog.

Superior Trading Co., 837 Washington St., San Francisco, California 94108.
  You must write and request a catalog and let them know what you want. They sell ginseng, and herbs are listed in Chinese characters.

Taylor's Herb Garden Inc., 1535 W. Lane Oak Rd., Vista, California 92083.
Wonderful herbs, reasonably priced and many are difficult to obtain otherwise.

Tillotson's Roses, Brown's Valley Rd., Watsonville, California 95076. Old roses and new roses, fragrant, lovely roses. Send for the beautiful descriptive catalog.

Whole Herb Co., 250, E. Blitherdale, Mill Valley, California.
A nice shop with both wholesale and retail departments. Sells herbs, books, ginseng, etc. Mail-order catalog 25¢.

Williams-Sonoma, P. O. Box 3792, San Francisco, California 94119 for mail-order, and 576 Sutter St., San Francisco, California.
Exquisite cooking goodies including *pain de mie* for rectangular breads, black steel baguette and quiche pans.

COLORADO

Walter Drake & Sons, Drake Bldg., Colorado Springs, Colorado 80940.
A few interesting cooking items are listed in the mail-order catalog; Revere 1-cup saucepan just the ticket for a single person. Mail-order.

Green Mountain Herbs, Ltd., P.O. Box 2369,   4890 Pearl Street,
Boulder, Colorado 80306. Mail-order.

CONNECTICUT

Capriland's Herb Farm, Silver St., Coventry, Connecticut 06238.
A fantastic place to visit and buy culinary herbs and seeds, herb tea, and many other things for the herb gardener. Make sure to make early reservations for a delicious meal. Mail-order.

Hemlock Hill Herb Farm, Litchfield, Connecticut 06759.
Grows and sells very good herbs. Mail-order.

Truc International, Inc., Box 167, Woodstock Hill, Connecticut 06281.
Wonderful jams and jellies made with herbs and many delightful herbal body care products. Mail-order catalog.

FLORIDA

Greyhound Gift House, 7178 NW 12th St., Miami, Florida 33126.
Some elegant kitchen items. Mail-order catalog.

Joan Cook, 853 Eller Dr., Ft. Lauderdale, Florida 33316.
All kinds of knicky-knacky things for the kitchen including small items for a small kitchen or for single persons.

GEORGIA

Kaleidoscope, 2201 Faulkner Rd. NE, Atlanta, Georgia 30324.
This is one of my favorite mail-order houses; quality good to superior; service often quick. Many elegant serving and kitchen goodies. Mail-order.

Sunnyland Farms, Albany, Georgia 31702.
Pecans plain and fancy. Mail order.

ILLINOIS

Downs, Dept. 176 and Dept. 476 for Collectors, Evanston, Illinois 60204.
Blue enamel cooking utensils, graniteware and other items. Mail-order.

Pfaelzer Brothers, 4501 West District Blvd., Chicago, Illinois 60632. Expensive pieces of meat. Mail-order.

Herbarium, Inc., 2019 West Iowa St., Chicago, Illinois 60622, or Rt. 2, Box 620, Kenosha, Illinois.
Imports and exports herbs. Wholesale mail-order.

INDIANA

Abbey Press, St. Meinrad, Indiana 47577.
Mostly Christian items but some nice baskets are shown. Mail-order.

Indiana Botanic Gardens, Hammond, Indiana 46325.
An excellent herb store with many exotic items seldom found elsewhere such as Vanilla oil. Mail-order.

KANSAS

Cook's Geranium Nursery, 712 North Grand, Lyons, Kansas 67554.
Sells all kinds of geranium plants (scented Pelargoniums). Mail-order.

KENTUCKY

Berea College, Student Craft Industries, Berea, Kentucky 40404. Many lovely hand-made objects such as brooms, egg cups, cutting boards, etc. Mail-order.

MASSACHUSETTS

Organic Food Cellar, 31 Putnam Ave., Cambridge, Massachusetts 02139.
Good selection.

The Country Loft, South Shore Industrial Park, Hingham, Massachusetts 02043.
Some nice items for the kitchen are in the mail-order catalog.

Seth & Jed's Country Store, Great Barrington, Massachusetts 01230.
Many nice things, full selection of Sabatier knives, cast-iron cookware (4½ qt. Dutch oven—$16.95), nice braided rugs for the kitchen, beautiful ceramic dishware with the exquisite Botanic Garden design. Mail-order.

MINNESOTA

Gokey's, 21 W. 5th St., Saint Paul, Minnesota 55102.
Many items including wild rice, butcher block, gourmet steamer, etc. Mail-order.

MISSOURI

Alewel's Meats, South St. Louis St., Concordia, Missouri 64020.
I have not tried their ham or bacon but it looks good. Old Missouri meat that is smoked and aged. Mail-order.

NEW HAMPSHIRE

Brookstone Company, 4 Vose Farm Rd., Peterborough, New Hampshire 03458. Lots of good and interesting stuff, unique tools, household and culinary items. Mailorder.

NEW JERSEY

New Hampton General Store, RFD, Hampton, New Jersey 08827.
Mail-order.

NEW MEXICO

Josie's Best Blue Corn Tortillas, 1731 2nd St., Santa Fe, New Mexico.
There are addresses in the tortilla section of the recipes in this book listing more blue corn sources.

NEW YORK

Anthroposophic Press, 258 Hungry Hollow Rd., Spring Valley, New York 10977.
Books dealing with anthroposophy. Get *Herbs in Nutrition* by Maria Geuter. Mail-order.

Aphrodisia, 28 Carmine St., New York, New York 10014.
An incredible array of goodies in an incredible store. Their mail-order catalog is well worth the $1.00 they ask for.

Caswell-Massey, Lexington Ave. & 48th St., New York, New York 10017. Catalog Dept., 320 West 13th St., New York, New York 10014.
A fantastic collection of cosmetics and products used in the kitchen. Do send for the catalog.

Colonial Garden Kitchens, 270 West Merrick Rd., Valley Stream, New York 11582.
All the neat little odds and ends, cookware, gourmet foods are listed in the catalog. Mail-order.

Hammacher Schlemmer, 147 East 57 St., New York, New York 10022. Many interesting cooking items are shown in the catalog which I originally got for the linen and cotton sheets they advertise. Mail-order.

Kiehl Pharmacy, 109 3rd Ave., New York, New York 10003.
Who could go to New York without visiting this marvelous place. Herbs and perfume oils and many other products. *Go there and see!* Oh, how I wish they had a mail-order department.

Lewis & Conger, 39-25 Skillman Ave., Long Island City, New York 11104.
Mail-order.

Paprikas Weiss Importer, 1546 2nd Ave., New York, New York 10028.
I love their catalog, and love looking at the goodies listed; enamelware, different kinds of honeys, books—the only thing that troubles me is that their prices seem very high. Mail-order.

Weleda, Inc., 30 South Main St., Spring Valley, New York 10977.
I have tried everything in their catalog and am impressed not only with the body-care products but with the elixirs that are used as an alterative for good health. Mail-order.

OREGON

Atlantis Rising, 7915 SE Stark, Portland, Oregon 97215.
An incredible herb catalog with lots of information. Mail-order.

Nichols Garden Nursery, 1190 North Pacific Highway, Albany, Oregon 97321.
A tremendous catalog full of seeds, basic ingredients, herb plants. Mail-order.

PENNSYLVANIA

Adam York, Unique Products Co., 340 Poplar St., Hanover, Pennsylvania 17331.
Some nice kitchen and serving things. Mail-order.

Penn Herb Company, 603 No. 2nd St., Philadelphia, Pennsylvania 19123.
A great catalog full of herbs, herb products and basics.

RHODE ISLAND

Meadowbrook Herb Garden, Wyoming, Rhode Island 02898. Wonderful culinary
herb mixtures, good books, essential oils, many kinds of tea balls, nonalcoholic
elixirs meant to be used as dietary supplements, tea mixtures and herbs and seeds
are all listed in the mail-order catalog.

SOUTH CAROLINA

Periculum, P. O. Box 6421, Columbia, South Carolina 29206.
Nice things including ceiling fans. Mail-order.

TENNESSEE

Early's Honey Stand, RR 2, Box 100, Spring Hill, Tennessee 37174.
Old-fashioned foods, delicious dry salt-cured and smoked hams (not those soggy
stuffed full-of-water hams you find in some supermarkets), bacon, sausage, cheese
and other Southern style goodies. Mail-order.

TEXAS

Ault Bee Farms, Weslaco, Texas 78596.
Honey and royal jelly and *Aloe vera* by the pound. Mail-order.

Hilltop Herb Farm, Box 866, Cleveland, Texas 77327.
From the reports I hear, this is truly a fantastic place; serving delicious meals, healthy
herb plants, books, and scented geraniums, and it is run by some of the most
wonderful people I have ever met. Mail-order catalog 30¢.

Horchow Collection, P. O. Box 34257, Dallas, Texas 75234.
An elegant catalog full of elegant items including many useful in the kitchen. Mail-
order.

VERMONT

Crowley Cheese, Healdville, Vermont 05147.
Cheese made solely from fresh whole milk without additives, preservatives or anything artificial. Mail-order.

Harrington's in Vt., Inc., Main Street, Richmond, Vermont 05477.
Smoked ham, bacon, turkey and game. Mail-order.

Swayze, Henry and Cornelia, Brookside Farm, Tunbridge, Vermont 05077.
Delicious, pure, wonderful maple syrup.

VIRGINIA

Byrd Mill Co., P. O. Box 5167, Richmond, Virginia 23220.
Real old-fashioned country hams and various food products like grits, mixes.
Mail-order.

Claiborne Johnston, 12 So. 3rd St., Richmond, Virginia 23205.
Various Virginia-style hams, bacons, and turkeys. Mail-order.

Hudson Ham House, Rt. 3, Box 27, Culpeper, Virginia.
Country cured hams, shoulders and sliced ham. Mail-order.

WISCONSIN

Figi's Inc., Marshfield, Wisconsin 54449.
Bulk cheeses and gift packages. Mail-order.

Wisconsin Cheese Makers Guild, 6048 West Beloit Rd., Milwaukee, Wisconsin 53219.
Bulk cheeses and gift packages. Mail-order.

The Soap Opera, 312 State St., Madison, Wisconsin 53703.
An excellent assortment of body care goodies including flower waters that are
pure and can be used in cooking.

CANADA

Wide World of Herb Ltd., 11 Saint Catherine Street East, Montreal, Canada 129.
Quebec.
So much is listed in this catalog, essential oils and herbs. An incredible combo.
Wholesale and retail mail-order.

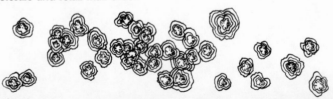

Part II

The Recipes

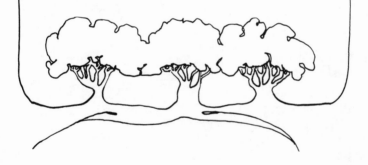

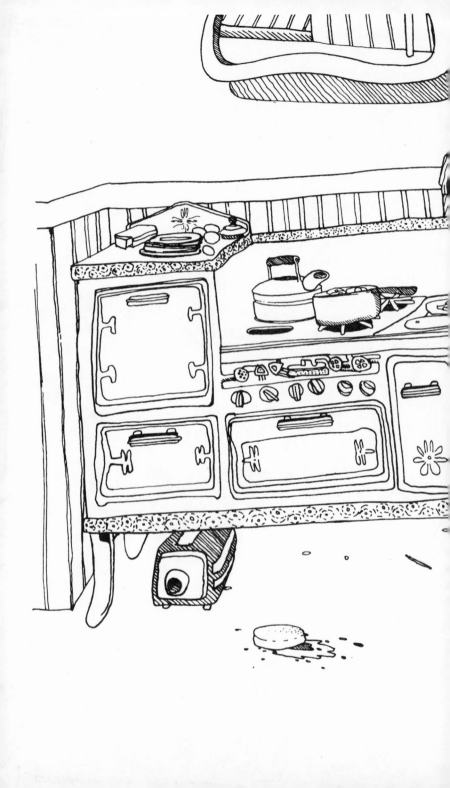

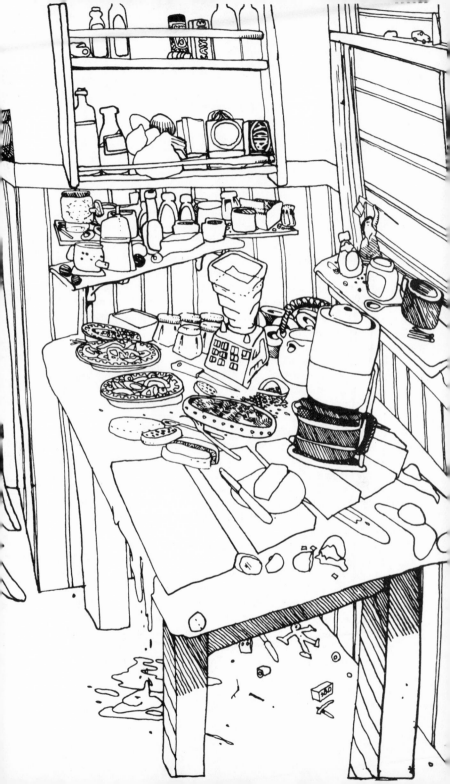

Chapter 7

A Fantastic Breakfast & Other Divine Devices

In early spring Michael and I decided that dinner parties were too exhausting but that a super brunch was just right. Since our usual breakfast consists of nothing for me, and yogurt and wheat germ mix for both Mike and boy Bryan, any special occasion calls for Eggs Benedict, or what I call Eggs Rosas. And a special occasion that calls for Eggs Rosas also calls for a house full of friends that, due to our demanding schedules, we hardly ever see. So, in early spring we organized three brunches. I would like to thank everyone who came to those late morning parties and helped me to experiment with various recipes, but a special thanks to the regulars who attended each one and who were able to make comparisons as to the style and content of each menu. So thanks Mac, Pam, Tom, and a special mention to our super-regular John, who helped me work off the effects of champagne after one party by wildly bicycling me around the park.

What did we eat? Our basic menu was a first course of champagne mixed with an equal amount of freshly squeezed Orange juice, served with a perfectly ripened Brie and various crackers. We stopped adding the Orange juice pulp after Pam decided that chewing Orange juice champagne cocktails was just not her favorite way of drinking a morning beverage. (You do know, of course, that it is very important to include pulp in your juice as well as some of the white membrane of the Orange because that is what contains the bioflavonoids, and you really do not get the benefit of Vitamin C without it.)

The next course was Eggs Rosas, which is similar to Eggs Benedict except for the substitution of different vegetables for the traditional piece of Canadian bacon. Twice, along with the Eggs Rosas, I served thin green spears of Asparagus. At the third breakfast we broke with tradition and had Artichokes with a special sauce. The wine with this second course was *Oiel de Perdrix,* from Sutter Home Winery in California. The third course consisted of a light dessert and a strong coffee, strong enough to stand by itself without a cup! Dessert ranged from delightful Madeleines (the very taste of which brought back such memories to Proust that an entire book was written) to other assorted sweets from our nearby Tassajara Bakery to Amaretti cookies from Italy.

And possibly the most important part of any party, whether it be brunch or cocktails, are the guests. They should be well-spoken and able to sit on the grass for at least four hours. We had all of Mike's local siblings, our court astrologer Jim, who reinvented Astral Astrology (Astro-Carto-Graphy), and the regulars, as well as an elegant pair of acquaintances from North Beach at Breakfast One. At Breakfast Two we had the doctor, the lawyer, and the architect, and, of course, the regulars. This is the party that I mostly forgot, rode wildly around the park, flying kites, seeing movies, eating ice cream, and forgetting just about everything, including how to cook. For this breach of manners and memories, I must now thank Penny, Terence, and John for getting me through it. At party three we had more longtime friends, the super-regulars, a pair of art historians, and the only person who smokes that I don't mind being around.

The next most important part of a party is being able to put together the ingredients in such a manner that nothing which is critical is forgotten, nothing burned nor neglected, and one in which all the parts come together at the right moment so that everyone is fed within a reasonable time. When serving Eggs Benedict or Eggs Rosas, this can be difficult. I suggest you set your table the night before, arrange flowers and lay out any serving pieces. Write down in advance everything you will need to do and the order in which you should do it. Try to buy all the groceries at least two days in advance. If you are making any special sauces that need a day or two to age, be sure to make them a day or two in advance. Decide what your accoutrements will be with the eggs and the proper herbs to go with them. Remove the eggs and butter from the fridge so they will be at room temperature when you get ready to use them in the morning. Make sure you have at least one bottle of wine per person chilling in the fridge (that is, for our guests who guzzle champagne and wine like a frog takes to water). Take an herb bath, wash your hair, get out your dream pillow, then go to bed.

If your party starts at 9:30 A.M., you will have guests arriving from 9 A.M. until 11 A.M. Get the early arrivals to squeeze the Orange juice, and let all the guests help themselves to the drinks, Brie, and crackers. It would also be nice to have a bowl of chilled fruit, such as Grapes and tiny Tangerines, and, when available, big, delicious Strawberries.

When all the guests have arrived and everyone is nicely loose and happy, start preparing the rest of the breakfast. Have the Artichokes cooked, cooled, cored, and stuffed, or the Asparagus started. The Hollandaise sauce is made in the blender with egg yolks, Tarragon-flavored vinegar or Lemon juice, and the hot butter is slowly dripped in. While you are making the Hollandaise, the water should be coming to a boil for the poached eggs (don't forget to add a bit of vinegar to the boiling water so the whites don't spread). Toast the sour-dough English muffins in the oven or toaster. Some folks precook the poached eggs so that everyone can eat at once, but we find that poaching eggs for three people at a time is just about right for getting fifteen people fed, talked, and happy in an hour's time. So, when the muffins are toasted and the Hollandaise done, drop 6 eggs, one at a time, in the gently simmering water.

Lightly butter the muffins and put them in the oven to keep warm. Grab a warm plate, put a serving of Asparagus or an Artichoke on it, 2 muffin halves, a choice of toppings on the muffins, and one poached egg on each muffin. Cover the lot with Hollandaise, sprinkle on the appropriate seasoning, and serve. Have a camera ready in case someone, due to exuberance, gracefully drops a poached egg sunnyside up, yolk unbroken, on the floor.

I have talked about vegetarian replacements that one can use on English muffins instead of the traditional Canadian bacon. My favorites are: sliced Tomatoes, sliced sweet Onions, sautéed Mushrooms with a bit of Parsley, Artichoke hearts, Salsa Verde #1 (see chapter 15), or sliced Avocadoes. Put one of these on the muffin, top it with a poached egg, some Hollandaise sauce, and then sprinkle on the appropriate herb. Basil is good with Tomato, Rosemary with Onion, Tarragon with Mushroom, Oregano with Artichoke hearts, Cumin or Cilantro with Salsa Verde, and salad herbs with Avocadoes.

I should mention that even though I am not normally a vegetarian, I serve only vegetarian meals to my guests to show them that meat and meat products are not really necessary at a meal. Vegetarians can eat elegantly as well as healthily.

BREAKFAST RECIPES

EGGS ROSAS

HOLLANDAISE SAUCE:

1 stick (4 oz.) butter	Juice of half a small Lemon
3 egg yolks	Tarragon

In a small saucepan slowly melt the butter over low heat. In a blender blend the egg yolks for 3 minutes, then add the Lemon juice, some Tarragon, and blend for another minute. With the blender on medium speed, slowly add the melted butter dribble by dribble. The sauce will slowly thicken, and within 5 minutes you will have a perfect Hollandaise to use on Asparagus, vegetables, or poached eggs. Covers 12 muffin halves.

POACHED EGGS:

In a medium-sized, shallow, curved saucepan add a bit of butter and 1½ inches of water; bring to a low simmering boil, adding a dash of vinegar to keep the whites of the eggs from spreading. Gently crack open and slowly add your room-temperature eggs one at a time to the gently simmering water. (A medium-sized pan can usually take 6 eggs without crowding.) Spoon hot water over the top of the egg to set it and remove eggs with a slotted spoon or spatula when they have cooked to your liking.

MUFFIN COVERS:

Have five or six bowls at the ready with five or six different ingredients. Have the proper herb seasoning standing near each bowl (see above).

Technique:

12 English muffin halves, toasted and
   buttered

On each muffin half, cover with desired muffin toppings, add a poached egg, ladle on some warm Hollandaise sauce, and sprinkle on the herb seasoning.

Serves 6.

FRESH FRUIT SYRUP FOR CREPES OR PANCAKES

Penny gave me these recipes for desserts because in our home we do not make nor eat them and in her home they do. She says, "I would rather eat my occasional sweets at brunch than at the end of an evening meal. This syrup is not too sugary, but makes everyone happy, especially in the summertime when Peaches and Berries are ripe and plentiful."

2 C. cut-up fruit (Peaches and Berries   ⅓ C. or more of honey
   are best, but a combo of Bananas
   and raisins is also good)

Pour honey over the fruit and cook until mixture comes to a minimal boil. Do not overcook or the fruit gets too juicy and mushy.

Serves 4.

RAINBOW EGGS
(FOR A CHILDREN'S BREAKFAST, LUNCH, OR DINNER)

In plenty of butter over low heat scramble some eggs softly, and season them generously with herbs, salt and pepper, or whatever taste the children like. Divide the eggs into as many portions as you have colors. Arrange the eggs in a wheel shape on a large round platter, keeping the colors separate by making spokes of Parsley, bacon strips, vegetable crudities, Asparagus, sliced Tomatoes, or other foods. The hub of the wheel can be of black or green olives.

Red Eggs—colour with Tomato paste or Beet powder
Yellow Eggs—colour with Curry powder, Saffron, or Turmeric
Green Eggs—colour with finely chopped Parsley, Chervil, or a paste of Parsley or Chervil
Blue Eggs—colour with a small quantity of cooked blue Cornmeal, mush, or grits

You could also decorate the rim of your wheel of rainbow eggs by using the appropriate colors in sliced vegetables. For example: Red—sliced Tomatoes, sweet Red Pepper, Pimento, or Radishes; Yellow—small baby Corn, yellow Peppers, or yellow Squash; Green—Green Peppers, Peas, sweet pickles, or Broccoli; Blue—small wedges of Red Cabbage that have been lightly sautéed in an iron pan, or marinated Eggplant.

THE FAMOUS ONE-EYED MONSTER EGG

Butter	Pimento, thinly sliced
1 slice Whole Wheat bread	Parsley or Chervil
1 egg	1 small black olive
	Capers or raisins, optional

Put butter in a small skillet, heat and add a slice of bread that has a round hole cut out of the center about as big as a fifty-cent piece. Crack an egg into the hole so that the yolk slides in and the white spreads out on the bread. Cook over a low heat until the white has set. You may or may not cover the pan, and you may or may not decide to turn the whole thing "over easy." To simulate the bloodshot eye of a monster, add very thin slices of Pimento to the white as it soaks into the bread. Season with a

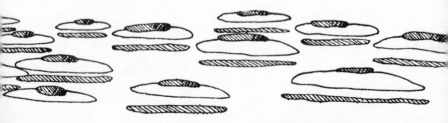

sprinkle of Parsley or Chervil, and add the olive to the center of the yolk for the pupil of the eye. You may add a caper or two, or a raisin, to approximate other monstrous eye abnormalities.

Serves 1.

MY MOMMA'S BREAD PUDDING

When my mom made bread pudding, she used dried up bread scraps that we had collected over a period of time. Mom never wasted anything, and I do not remember her using a recipe. When I had to recreate this recipe, I first had to feed my family quantities of sour dough bread before a sufficient number of crumbs and pieces were collected to begin the bread pudding experiment. Then, of course, my poor family had to eat bread pudding morning, noon, and night while I experimented with varying quantities of the ingredients. The following recipe is a *very* close approximation of the delicious dessert/breakfast food with which I grew up. It is much better to eat than any cold cereal, is very easy to make, and if it were analyzed, you would find that it contains everything that a normal human being needs to get going in the day.

3 eggs	1 C. raisins
4 C. (1 qt.) sweet milk or buttermilk	½ C. nut meats
1-inch piece of Cinnamon stick rubbed between the palms, or 1 t. Cinnamon powder	1 t. grated Lemon rind
	Dash of Cardamom
	8 C. bread cubes about 1-inch square (use old, dry bread)
1 C. dark Maple syrup (if you like things sweeter, make this 1½ C.)	Nutmeg

Mix together eggs, milk, Cinnamon, and Maple syrup. In a separate bowl combine the raisins, nuts, Lemon rind, Cardamom, and bread cubes, and mix together. Pour the egg mixture over the bread mixture and soak for 2 hours, or cover and refrigerate overnight. Put in a greased pan, sprinkle generously with Nutmeg, and bake in a preheated 325°F. oven for 40 minutes. Serve slightly warm or cool—and eat!

About 8 servings.

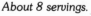
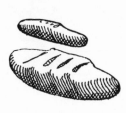
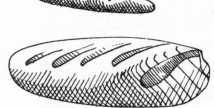

CREAM WITH RICE

A VERY good Cream to eat hot, is thus made. Into a quart of sweet Cream, put a spoonful of very fine powder of Rice, and boil them together sufficiently, adding Cinnamon, or Mace and Nutmeg to your liking. When it is boiled enough take it from the fire, and beat a couple of yolks of new-laid eggs, to colour it yellow. Sweeten it to your taste. Put bread to it in its due time.

A GOOD DISH OF CREAM

Boil a quart of good Cream with sticks of Cinnamon and quartered Nutmeg and Sugar to your taste. When it is boiled enough to have acquired the taste of the Spice, take the whites of six New laid eggs, and beat them very well with a little Fresh cream, then pour them to your boyling Cream, and let them boil a walm* or two. Then lit it run through a boulter,** and put a little Orange flower water to it, and sliced bread; and so serve it up cold.
                                        —*The Closet of Sir Kenelm Digbie Knight Opened*

BUCKWHEAT CAKES OR WAFFLES

When I visited my great-uncle Ed in Canada some years ago, the season was winter and the weather was extremely cold. My uncle spent the greater part of the evenings regaling me with extremely obscene jokes in Canadian patois. Fortunately for me, my French was very poor and it was quite sometime before I understood the words in these jokes. In the mornings, however, after he showered and rolled in the snow, he would make absolutely delicious buckwheat pancakes with just flour, water and oil on his woodburning stove. Our adventures out into the world to get this Buckwheat flour, that could only be obtained from a certain little store in a particular little village, were quite memorable. I have lost his exact recipe in the morass of my brain's storage banks, but the taste and scent of those delicious cakes served with head cheese and Maple syrup will stay with me to the end of my days. Uncle Ed said that Buckwheat cakes and Maple syrup would cure any ailment if eaten with a right and peaceful heart—and I believe him.

2 t. dry yeast (activated granular)	2 T. Corn oil
1 C. lukewarm water	3 C. water, milk, or a mix of both
2 T. honey or Maple syrup	2 C. Buckwheat flour
1 C. Buckwheat flour	1 t. salt

Soften the yeast in the water, add the sweet and the 1 cup Buckwheat flour, mix it all together and set aside until nice and bubbly, about 1 hour. In a large bowl

*walm is a boiling up.
**boulter probably means some sort of sifter or strainer.

mix together the oil and water or milk. Mix together the rest of the flour and salt and add to the milk. Add the yeast mixture and beat together. Cover with a clean cloth, set in a warm place, let it rise (about 2 hours), give it another stir with a wooden spoon, and then bake as pancakes or waffles.

3—6 servings.

ROSE PETAL SCRAMBLED EGGS

20—25 Red Rose petals	Bacon, cooked (about 3 slices per
6 eggs	person)
A little water	Tarragon
	English muffins, toasted

Pick Roses in the morning before the sun has been able to dry out their volatile oils. Gently wash the Rose petals, dry them by draining on a paper towel, cut off and discard the white tip which is very bitter, and sliver the petals with a sharp knife. Beat and scramble the eggs with the water, adding a very delicate touch of Tarragon. Add the Rose petal slivers to the cooked eggs, and serve with bacon and muffins.

Variations:

Omelets and scrambled eggs can also be made with Violet flowers, Mullein flowers, Nasturtiums, and other flowers that have a pronounced flavor.

Serves 3.

BLUE-CORN ATOLE

Blue corn has a more corny flavor than yellow corn, and when it cooks it turns the most delightful psychedelic purple color. It is absolutely divine in tortillas and makes a superior tasting *atole*. You can get Blue cornmeal from El Encanto Mexican Foods; 1224 Airway Drive, SW; Albuquerque, New Mexico; 87105. Ask for Harina de Maiz made from Indian blue corn.

½ C. cold water	2 C. boiling water with ¼ t. salt added
½ C. blue Cornmeal (other Cornmeal	Warm milk
can be substituted)	Cinnamon, Cumin, Nutmeg, or any
	other tasty spice

Mix the Cornmeal into the cold water. Add this slowly to the boiling water. Cook until the mixture is creamy and smooth, about 5 minutes. Pour into mugs and fill only half or three-quarters full. Fill the mug with warm milk. Sprinkle this delicious, healthful drink with Cinnamon, Cumin, Nutmeg, or other spice. A dollop of honey may be added, if desired.

Serves 2—3.

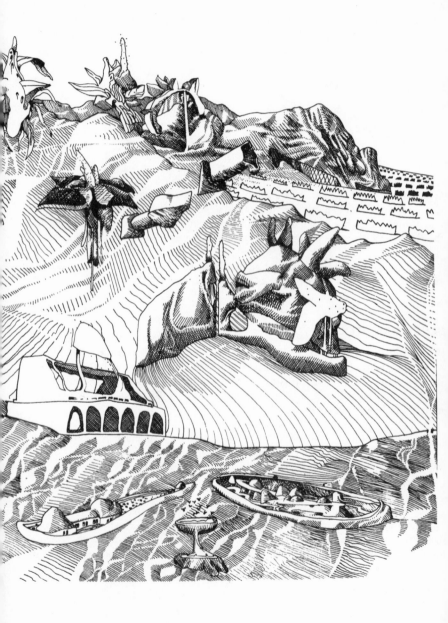

Chapter 8

The Garlic Lunch or 101 Ways to Eat a Taco or Use a Tortilla

THE TORTILLA VENDOR

He who sells . . . tortillas, sells thick ones and thin ones. Some are round, . . . some are filled . . . some are folded-over tortillas . . . some are large and thin . . . some are large and thick . . . ; tortillas cooked in the coals; tortillas made of Amaranth seeds and of ground Squash seeds and of green Corn and of Prickly Pears. Some of these are cooked, others toasted; some are cold, others hot.

—Fray Bernardino de Sahagun,
*Historia General de las Cosas de Nueva
Espana,* Book X, Chapter XVIII, late 16th century

"What is a tortilla? A round, thin 'pancake' of unleavened corn dough that has been prepared and eaten in Mexico from the earliest times until the present day. Parched corn kernels are briefly cooked in a solution of unslaked lime and water and then left to soak until they are soft enough to be ground to a smooth dough, or masa."

—from *The Tortilla Book,* a wonderful fantastic
no-nonsense, delicious eating cookbook written
by Diana Kennedy

TORTILLAS AND SOME TACO MIXTURES

Some years ago when Michael and I were still trying to devise a lunch for him that would be wholesome, but not contribute to his already nervous stomach, I happened to read an article in a magazine about Corn. The article explained that if you ate Corn as tortillas, not only would you be getting a healthy amount of lime in your diet, which contains Calcium, a nerve soother, but you also would have a means of excreting harmful strontium from your body. It seems that strontium from the atmosphere is absorbed daily into our systems and is constantly poisoning our body cells. When it combines with the calcium in the tortilla, an insoluble salt is formed that can then be harmlessly excreted.

If you examine the diet of the Aztecs, you will find that they were eating balanced, nutritious foods that combine perfectly.

Corn plus lime equal a tortilla and provide Calcium.
Corn plus Beans equal a perfectly balanced protein.
Chiles contain enormous amounts of Vitamins C and A.
Garlic is a natural anti-bacterial substance.
Squash contains much Vitamin A and is a source of many minerals.
Tomatoes contain Vitamins C and A.
Avocadoes, Sage, and the many other vegetables and herbs they ate contain other
   necessary nutrients.

We soon began to eat tortillas daily, starting by buying horrible, yellow-dyed stuff from the local market. Soon we realized our error and switched to the luscious, tender, just-made tortillas from local tortillarias. We devised many exotic tacos (which are tortillas stuffed with goodies) from these tortillas, and have found that anything is possible with these divine flat breads.

To Cook the Tortilla:
You must have a *comal* or a small cast-iron skillet to cook a tortilla. Coat the pan with a good quality Corn oil as it gives the resulting product a more Corny taste. I also like to use Blue Corn tortillas as often as possible. Heat your skillet, add the Corn oil, and swirl the pan to coat it. Toast one side of the tortilla, turn it over, put some shredded cheese to melt on the cooked side, and fold in half. When the cheese has melted and the outer side is somewhat toasted, remove from the griddle or skillet and fill with any number of goodies that you have placed in bowls on the table.

To Make the Taco:
Stuff it with anything handy, such as:

1. Avocado, sliced Garlic, String Cheese, Mayonnaise, Sprouts
2. Avocado, sliced Garlic, Cheese, Shrimp, Salsa
3. Shredded Cooked Chicken, Cheese, Salsa
4. Shrimp, Salsa, Sprouts
5. Tomatoes, Cheese, Mayonnaise
6. Beans, Cheese, Sprouts, Salsa
7. Black Beans, Epasote, Lettuce, Salsa
8. Avocado, sliced Garlic, Chili, Sprouts, Cilantro

9. My favorite: Avocado, Garlic pieces, Provolone, Shrimp, freshly grown Alfalfa Sprouts, Cilantro
10. Avocado, Chili, Muenster, Onions
11. Tomato, Eggs, Cilantro, Sprouts
12. Chicken, Sour Cream, sliced Garlic, Tomatoes, Chili
13. Crab, Sour Cream, sliced Garlic, Sprouts, Lemon juice
14. Mushrooms, sliced Garlic, Avocado, Sprouts, Salsa

The list, of course, is endless and can be improvised upon, depending on what you have available in your refrigerator. You can use any kind of leftovers: from meats, to dips, to chopped vegetables. We always like to have some kind of cheese in our tacos and, of course, the ubiquitous Garlic—though it has earned us some kind of reputation with our local dentist. (He now only makes appointments with us in the morning and *not* after lunch.)

To Eat the Taco:
Invite all your friends over so that they will all have the same Garlic breath. Take the tortilla shell, stuff as previously described, bend over a plate, and eat, bite by bite, each luscious morsel of the taco. Have two or three tacos, some tasty tea, and you will feel revitalized and renewed for the rest of the day.

Blue Corn Tortillas

First, obtain some Blue Corn. Order it or drive to New Mexico. (Bueno Food Products, 1224 Airway Dr., S.W. Albuquerque, New Mexico 87105). I feel that Blue Corn makes the most delicious, certainly the most colorful Corn tortilla possible.

To make Blue Corn tortillas with Blue *Harina de Maiz,* just add a pinch of salt, and a pinch of baking powder for leavening, if preferred, to one cup of *Harina de Maiz.* Add enough water to the mixture so that you are able to shape the dough into small round cakes, and flatten using a rolling pin. Place on a hot, greased comal (griddle) until done. Cover with Salsa, stuff with Avocadoes and shrimp, do any of the 10,001 + 1 things you can do with a cooked tortilla, and you have a delicious, nutritious meal.

SQUASH BLOSSOM QUESADILLA IN RED

1 tortilla
Some grated cheese

Red Nasturtium blossoms, chopped
Red Salsa
Squash blossoms, chopped
Hot Red Peppers, chopped

Fold the tortilla in half, put all the ingredients inside, and fry each side in Corn oil until browned. Cover with red Salsa and eat. Use ingredients to taste.

Variation in Yellow:

1 tortilla
Armenian string cheese
Squash blossoms, chopped
Garlic, chopped

Hot Yellow Peppers, chopped
Minced Onions
Pinch of Epasote
Yellow Chili sauce

Fold the tortilla in half, put all the ingredients inside, and fry each side in Corn oil until browned. Cover with yellow Chili sauce.

Serves 1.

Chapter 9

Soup & Salad, the Basic Dinner

"I *WILL* get some worms and go fishing and catch a dish of minnows for my dinner," said Mr. Jeremy Fisher. "If I catch more than five fish, I will invite my friends Mr. Alderman Ptolemy Tortoise and Sir Isaac Newton. The Alderman, however, eats salad."

The Tale of Mr. Jeremy Fisher
by Beatrix Potter

(AND Mr. Alderman Ptolemy Tortoise brought a salad with him in a string bag.)

SOUPS

THE GARLIC ROSE

"You are what you eat" and "Let food be your medicine" are always easy things to say, but these deathless lines are rarely backed up with any concrete information about what one *should* eat or how to prepare it. As a member of the board of directors of the "Lovers of the Stinking Rose," an organization dedicated to that most wonderful of foods, GARLIC, it was my pleasure to devise recipes using Garlic both as a food and as a medicine. This particular recipe for Garlic Soup is excellent food for an invalid, especially one suffering from digestive problems, bacterial infection, or respiratory difficulty. It can act as a vermifuge when eaten in quantity over a period of a few days. If you add Cayenne or another Chile, this delicious dish will quickly open a stuffy nose and help clear a blocked bronchial condition.

Children will love this soup; Garlic-haters, unaware of what is in it, will also love it. Learn how to make this easy soup; eat it frequently. You will find your health, well-being, and internal and external beauty will improve, and the flu season will come and go without your suffering even a little bit. As the herbalist John Parkinson said in 1629 in his fantastic *Paradisi in Sole Paradisus terrestris:*

> It being well boyled in falt broth, is often eaten of them that haue ftrong ftomackes, but will not brooke in a weake and tender ftomacke. It is accounted, and fo called in diuers Countries, The poore mans Treacle, that is, a remedy for all difeafes. It is neuer eaten rawe of any man I know, as other of the rootes aforefaid, but sodden alwaies and fo taken. Ranfoms are oftentimes eaten with bread and butter, and otherwife alfo, as euery mans affection and courfe of life leadeth him to vfe . . . .

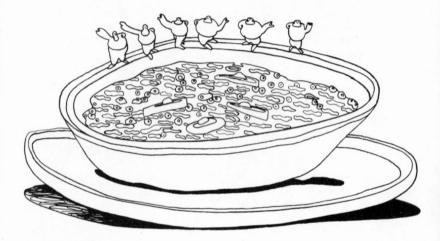

GARLIC SOUP

2–40 Garlic cloves (about 1–4 bulbs)
2 T. or more good quality Olive oil

1 qt. rich chicken or vegetable broth or stock
3 egg yolks
Chopped Parsley, Yogurt, ground Almonds, optional

Crush the Garlic cloves with the flat of a knife and slip off skins. Sauté the Garlic slowly in oil in a cast-iron skillet until translucent. Add the broth or stock (that means liquid only, no solids or blended foods), and simmer gently about 20 minutes until the Garlic is mushy. Press the Garlic-broth blend through a ricer or sieve, or squeeze through coarse cheesecloth into a bowl. Beat the egg yolks until thick with a wire whisk in a two-quart enamelware or stainless steel pot. Then beat in slowly, a teaspoon at a time, some of the warm Garlic broth. Beat in about 3 T. all together. (What we are trying to do here is warm up the egg yolks without cooking them.) Combine the two mixtures slowly, heat to boiling, and serve in wide soup plates.

This soup can be a delicious first course of a meal—just add dollops of chopped Parsley, Yogurt, and ground Almonds to the soup when it is served.

The soup is mainly seasoned by the broth. If desired, add any of the following depending on the results you wish to obtain: salt, Pepper, Cayenne, Oregano, or Parsley.

Once I served this soup as a first course to a group of people at a party. There was a confirmed Garlic-hater among us who swore that he could always tell when even the most miniscule amount of Garlic had been used in a food. He was well into his second bowl of soup when I asked him what kind of soup he thought it was. He guessed it to be a rich Leek soup. When I denied that and said it was 40-Clove Garlic Soup, his face blanched and he immediately stopped eating.

Serves 4−6.

MELINDA'S CHRISTMAS TOMATO SOUP

There are a lot of "Moores" in Mike's family and when we were all gathered together at Christmas, Grammy had a lot of cooking to do. One year she came up with a delightful, novel and ego-fulfilling idea about cooking. We all chose lots and two of us each night planned a meal, shopped, cooked, served, ate, and did the dishes. We were each able to do our best recipes. Mindy's soup is not your usual watery, no-personality soup. It is rich and delicious, and when served with sour-dough bread and a giant salad it is a most satisfying meal.

24 medium to large Tomatoes, really ripe and juicy
2 t. sugar, optional
1 stick (¼ lb.) butter
1 or 2 Onions, sliced and coarsely chopped
2 crushed Bay leaves
3−6 Celery stalks with the tops coarsely chopped

1 T. or more minced sweet Basil (or Korean Mint for a different flavor)
1 t. salt
1/4 t. Peppercorns crushed in a mortar (Szechuan pepper is nice here)
1/2 bunch chopped Parsley with stalks
1 Lemon, scrubbed, juiced, sliced
1−5 Garlic cloves, sliced

Mix all together in a cast-iron Dutch oven and simmer over a very low heat 4−6 hours. Stir occasionally. Excellent also with a vegetable salad and a quiche.

Serves 4−8.

A GOOD VEGETARIAN VEGETABLE SOUP AND STOCK

Dedicated to Joe Carcione who said, "One Leek in a pot of soup goes a long way."

Some Italian Olive oil
5 Garlic cloves, crushed
2 large Leeks, sliced
5 Carrots, sliced
2 large Potatoes, halved and sliced
3 stalks Celery, sliced, with tops

1 T. soup herbs (see Chapter 17)
1 T. chopped Chervil
1 T. salt, Celery salt, or Kelp
1 qt. good hearty burgundy
5 Tomatoes, quartered
2 qt. water
1 large handful Parsley, chopped

In a cast-iron Dutch oven, heat the Olive oil, and add the Garlic, Leeks, Carrots, Potatoes, Celery, soup herbs, Chervil, and salt. Sauté at medium high heat until the Potatoes are slightly browned. Add the wine and bring to a boil. Immediately add the water, Tomatoes, and the Parsley. Cover and simmer 1–2 hours. Eat the soup, or let it rest overnight to age, reheat, and eat it the next day. You can also strain out the vegetables and eat them with a generous sprinkling of Parmesan cheese, and then use the liquid as soup stock or broth. The stock is delicious as a base for the Garlic Soup, especially if you are a vegetarian and adverse to using a chicken stock. The vegetables are so soft that they are an excellent food for babies or invalids. In any case this delicious soup can be used many ways. I have also used the stock, thinned with an equal amount of hot water, as a broth when I am fasting. It is very nourishing and filling to the stomach. Add a really generous amount of Cayenne Pepper to the broth, heat it until hot, eat, and it makes an exceedingly delicious medicine to help clear out plugged sinuses.

Serves 4–8.

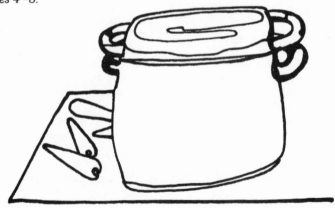

MY FIFTH VEGETABLE SOUP

I have a friend who quite casually suggested that I try vegetarianism. He made the point that for someone who lectured as much as I did about the virtues of the diet, I should at least try it or stop talking about it. So I did, but it was somewhat difficult. I am the product of a French mother and had never before tried to make soup without at least a delicious marrow bone. The first soups I tried were okay, but this one was delicious, although the ingredients may seem a little bit odd.

1 red Onion, sliced	1 bottle (3–4 C.) hearty burgundy
4 or more Garlic cloves, whole and peeled	1–2 qt. water
Celery tops, chopped	1 Tomato, quartered
1 Sweet Potato, halved and sliced	Small handful Calendula petals
2 Carrots, sliced	Spices: 1 t. Korean Mint, crushed
Some sliced Cabbage	½ t. crushed Coriander seeds
1 green hot Chile Pepper, sliced	1 piece (1–2 inches) Cinnamon stick
Olive oil	1 T. All-Purpose Herb Blend (see Chapter 17)

Sauté all the vegetables together in some Olive oil until the potato is slightly browned. Add the hearty burgundy, water, Tomato, Calendula, and the spices. Simmer together for an hour. Let age and meld for a few hours or overnight before reheating and serving. You may want to add some Dulse, Kelp, or salt before serving. This soup is delicious with some sour-dough French bread and a huge, delicious vegetable salad.

Serves 4–8.

A JOY OF A BLACK BEAN SOUP

1 lb. black Beans	5 T. Olive oil
2 qt. water	2 medium Onions, chopped
1 ham hock, optional	2 Green Peppers, chopped
5 Garlic cloves	Garnish:
2 T. salt	1 raw Onion, chopped or chopped green Onions
1½ t. Cumin, ground	1 t. Olive oil
1½ t. Oregano, crushed	½ t. vinegar
Leaf or two Epazote	

Soak the black Beans overnight. Drain them and put into a kettle with 2 quarts of water and the ham hock (the hock is optional). Simmer and cook until the beans are tender, about 2–4 hours depending on the age of the beans. Crush together the Garlic cloves, salt (less than 2 T. if using the ham hock), Cumin, Oregano, and Epazote. Heat the Olive oil in a saucepan. Stir in the Onions, Green Peppers, and the Garlic mixture. Stir in 1 t. water, and simmer until the Onions are tender, about 5–10 minutes. Add this Onion mixture to the Beans and simmer until the flavours are well combined.

Garnish:

In a separate bowl marinate the chopped raw Onion or the green Onions in the Olive oil and vinegar.

To serve, pour the soup into bowls and garnish.

Serves 4–8.

Contributed by Joy Lippincott.

SPLIT PEA SOUP

This is Amber's favorite soup when it is hot, and it is my favorite dip, with Chile added, when it is cold.

1 C. split Peas (that have been soaked overnight)	1 Onion, well chopped
Water	1–5 cloves Garlic
1 piece salt pork, old fashioned salted, smoked bacon, or a ham bone	Olive or Safflower oil
	Pinch of dry Mustard
	Pinch of hot Red Pepper

In a soup pot add the split Peas (that have been soaked overnight) and water to twice the depth of the Peas. Add the salt pork, bacon, or ham bone. In a skillet lightly sauté Onions and Garlic until slightly browned. (Use Olive oil or Safflower oil depending on the taste you prefer.) Add the sautéed Onion and Garlic to the Peas in the pot, plus a goodly pinch of the Mustard and a small pinch of the Red Pepper. Stir occasionally as the soup simmers for the next few hours, and add water as needed. Simmer until tender and mushy. Peas are flowers, and so to have a complete protein you need to combine Pea Soup with a grass, such as a sprout salad or Whole Wheat bread. Your soup seasonings can be salt, Curry powder, Thyme, Savory, Bay leaf, Celery tops, and/or Parsley.

Serves 4–8.

SUPER AVOCADO SUPPER SOUP

A delicious dish that is easy to make, attractive to serve, and very economical. It has everything in it to please even the most finicky of eaters.

Chicken Broth:

1 chicken	1 Bay leaf
Water to cover (2–3 qts.)	1 Onion, whole
1 T. salt or herb salt	2 Celery stalks with leaves
	2 Garlic cloves

Put all ingredients into a deep soup pot and simmer until the chicken is done. Remove the chicken, strip the meat from the bones and cut into large pieces. Cool and refrigerate. Strain and refrigerate the broth. (Save the bones for a soup stock to be used another day.)

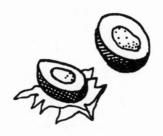

The Soup:

Chicken broth	3 small Potatoes, scrubbed and cut in half
6 Scallions or Spring Onions, whole	
3 ears of Corn, broken in half	6 flowerets of Broccoli or other green vegetable
3 large Carrots, sliced in half lengthwise	2 hearts of Celery with leaves, quartered
	3 large, ripe Avocadoes

Before serving, bring the broth to a boil, add all the vegetables, and cook until they are tender, about 15–20 minutes. Peel and halve the Avocadoes. Put them into 6 large, shallow soup bowls. Divide the vegetables equally among the bowls. Ladle the soup over the Avocado and vegetables. Serve with a sprinkle of soup herbs (Chapter 17) and a garnish of Parsley.

Serves 6.

UNCLE CYRILLE'S SOUP

My uncle makes a super vegetable soup. His secret, if there is one, is that he picks vegetables in season fresh from his garden. He has no herb garden, so for seasoning he takes a pinch of this and a pinch of that from some ancient cans of herbs and spices he has sitting dead and dormant against the wall over the stove. This is probably the least desirable spot in the entire house to store seasonings because the heat of the stove causes almost instant deterioration of the magical green seasonings. However, Uncle Cy's soup is souper and we all love it.

5 Garlic cloves, chopped	1 small green Bell Pepper, cut into
1 cracked soup bone	1-inch pieces
2 Onions, chopped	2 stalks Celery with the top leaves
Water to cover	chopped up
½ C. Rice or a chopped up Potato	3 Tomatoes, whole
6 small Carrots, cut into 1-inch pieces	1 t. salt
	Herbs of choice
	Butter
	1 T. dried Calendula petals

Put the Garlic, soup bone, and Onions into a soup pot, add water to cover and then some, and simmer for 5 hours. Add the remaining vegetables and the salt to the soup, and simmer until the vegetables are done. Sauté some herbs in a bit of butter. This is where Uncle Cy uses this and that, but you could start with Thyme, Rosemary, Basil, Oregano, or Marjoram, Bay leaf, Cloves, and Sage. Add the herbs to the soup. Then add the dried Calendula petals. Steep the herbs for a few minutes before serving. You can eat the soup in wide soup plates with a garnish of chopped Parsley.

Variation:

An alternate herbal mixture is a pinch of Thyme, 1 sprig Sage, 1 sprig Anise, Hyssop or Korean mint, 2 Camomile blossoms, and 1 T. dried Calendula petals.

Serves 4–8.

PUMPKIN SOUP

1 medium Pumpkin	6 egg yolks, beaten
Salt	Freshly ground black Pepper
½ C. heavy cream	Croutons
(Exact quantities depend on the size of the pumpkin.)	

Peel and clean the pumpkin, and cut into 1-inch cubes. Brown well over medium heat in a little salt (no oil) in an iron skillet. Cook in a covered pot until tender. Then purée pumpkin in a blender with the cream. Heat gently; add the egg yolks; heat through but do not boil. Season with pepper and croutons. Try serving the soup in a hollowed out pumpkin.

Serves 4–8.

MINESTRONE SOUP

3 qts. water
Bones (neckbones sautéed in Olive oil
1 C. Kidney or Garbanzo Beans
1 t. salt
1–4 cloves Garlic, minced
¼ t. black Pepper
1 large handful Parsley, chopped
1 T. Olive oil
1 Bay leaf
2 stalks Celery with tops, chopped

4 leaves Chard, chopped
1 small Zucchini, washed, unpeeled, and chopped
1 Carrot, scrubbed and chopped
1 Onion, chopped
2 green Onions, chopped
6 or more ripe Tomatoes, whole
1 bottle (3–4 C.) red wine
Water as needed to make soup the desired consistency
¼ C. macaroni

Simmer the bones and Beans in water until the Beans are tender. Remove the bones, and chill the soup. Remove the layer of fat from the chilled soup, and add the boned meat to this gelatinous soup base. Put the soup base and the boned meat in a large soup kettle and add the salt, Garlic, Pepper, Parsley, Olive oil, and Bay leaf. Simmer the mixture for about 20 minutes. Add the vegetables and simmer another hour. Add the wine, water, and macaroni, and simmer until the macaroni is tender, about 15 minutes. Serve the soup with grated Parmesan or Romano cheese, some chopped Basil, a loaf of good Garlic bread, and a nice crisp garden salad.

Serves 4–8.

DRIED CORN INDIAN SOUP

1 C. dried Corn, coarsely ground through a hand mill
Water enough to cover twice
1 piece smoked or salted bacon (the old fashioned kind), or salt pork
Garlic, crushed and peeled

Onion, sliced and chopped
Pepper
3 Juniper berries
Dash of Cayenne
1 T. Maple syrup
Salt, if necessary

Soak the Corn overnight in a heavy pot, and then bring it to a boil. Skim off the foam and turn down the fire so that the mixture just simmers. Sauté the bacon in a frying pan until a little fat collects. Add the Onions, Garlic, Pepper, Cayenne, and Juniper berries, and sauté until the Onion is soft. Add the contents of the frying pan and the Maple syrup to the simmering Corn, and cook until the Corn is tender. As the soup thickens, add water or meat juices to keep the desired consistency.

Serves 4−6.

SALADS

A FLOWER SALAD

We must thank a truly lovely and serene lady who gave me this recipe, Denni McCarthy. She invited me to her house once for dinner when I was lecturing in her area. The dinner was a marvel, a delicious repast of simple, lovely, wholesome raw foods. This is the salad exactly as she wrote the recipe:

"On a round tray or plate create a beautiful circle of flowers, laying Lettuce, Chard or Comfrey leaves as a base. Begin from the center with a small mound of grated Red Cabbage; circle this with a border of Cauliflower chopped into tiny pieces followed by Broccoli bits and then a ring of Alfalfa Sprouts. Surround all this with the orange and yellow of sun-warmed Nasturtiums. Then gather some other edible flowers of the season: Borage with its cooling blue, Sweet Honeysuckle, hot Mustard and Radish flowers, the fragrant Violets, Rose Petals, Wild Onion, Sage, Thyme, Rosemary and Calendula. Sprinkle these in a loving way over the vegetables keeping the rhythm of the circle, growing from the center into a new creation, a new flower.

"In eating flowers we partake of the more refined essence of the plant; the final stage before returning to seed and completing the cycle of plant life. So the flower offers a more subtle energy, as well as sweet nectar. It has been said that flowers can speak to us and contain special healing powers. To gather and make this salad is one way of being with flowers and learning how they express the harmony of nature."

Well, Denni, all I can say is amen to that.

ROMAN SALAD

1 part Gruyère cheese
1 part Celery

1 part Mushrooms, raw and finely
   sliced
1/2 part Parsley, coarsely chopped
Vinaigrette dressing
Dijon mustard

Thinly slice on the diagonal the Celery, and julienne or sliver the Gruyère. Combine with the mushrooms and parsley and toss them together gently. Toss again with a vinaigrette dressing that has had a dollop of Dijon mustard added to it. Set aside the salad and let it rest for at least 30 minutes before serving so that the flavors blend. We like to do this salad early in the day and let it chill, covered, in the refrigerator until dinner time. Sometimes we also like to add an equal part of french-cut Green Beans cooked *al dente* and a sprinkle of Basil to the salad.

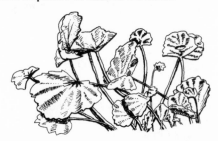

NASTURTIUM SALAD

1 large handful young Nasturtium leaves	Some Watercress
	Some Sprouts
1 large handful Lettuce leaves	3 or 4 Spring Onions, sliced diagonally

Wash the salad greens, roll in a clean towel, and refrigerate for a few hours. Then take the greens and tear them into bite-size pieces into a bowl. Add the Watercress, Sprouts, and the Spring Onions.

Dressing:	Salt
Salad oil (Olive and Safflower)	Pepper
Lemon juice	Marigold petals
Honey	Some Nasturtium flowers

Shake over the salad some oil (to taste, probably about ¼ C.), and toss lightly. Mix together the rest of the dressing ingredients (about ⅛ C.), and shake over the salad, and again toss lightly. Decorate with the Nasturtium flowers. Yum, yum. It has a delicious, fresh, slightly hot flavor. This salad is very good when served as an accompaniment to a bland main course, such as Mushrooms on toast. The salad is excellent as a cleanser for the liver.

Serves 4.

GREEK SALAD

1 Cucumber, peeled and sliced
2 Tomatoes, washed and cut into eighths
1 or 2 green Bell peppers, seeded and cut into strips
1 large sweet Spanish onion, peeled and thinly sliced
Greek Olives
1/2 lb. feta cheese, cut into 1/2-inch pieces

Greek Olive oil
a mixture of Lemon juice and red wine
salt
Pepper
1–3 Garlic cloves, crushed and peeled
1–3 T. crushed dried Oregano or Marjoram or a small handful of the fresh herb, chopped

Prepare the vegetables as directed and add the Olives and cheese. Mix the Olive oil, Lemon juice, red wine, salt, Pepper, and Garlic. There should be twice as much oil as acid (Lemon juice and wine), and enough of both to make a very generous dressing for the salad. Pour the dressing over the salad, toss, and add the Oregano. Refrigerate until needed.

This salad is especially good after it has aged in the refrigerator for a few hours or overnight. And now is the time to say that Olive oil tastes different when grown in different countries. You cannot make a real Greek-tasting salad by using California Olives and Olive oil. You must use the real thing. Try shopping at a Greek deli, or mail-order some by using the addresses in Chapter 6, pg. 118 for authentic ingredients. Greek Olive oil has an indefinable something that makes it perfect for Cucumbers, Onions, and Bell Peppers. Italian Olive oil, however, is perfect for pasta and to extract the essential oil of sweet flowers.

Serves 4–8.

MEXICAN-STYLE GREEK SALAD

1 lb. Zucchini, sliced and slightly cooked (sauté in a bit of Olive oil)
4 oz. Monterey Jack cheese, cubed
2 green Chiles, peeled and sliced
1 Avocado, sliced and cubed

1 small handful chopped Chives, or sliced Spring Onions or chopped Garlic to taste
1 stalk Celery, diagonally sliced
Romaine Lettuce
Pimento-stuffed green Olives

Combine the Zucchini, cheese, Chiles, Avocado, Chives (or alternative), and Celery.

Dressing:

1 Garlic clove, crushed	Salt
1/2 C. Spanish Olive oil	Pepper
1/4 C. mixture of Lemon juice and Tarragon vinegar	Generous pinch of Salad Herbs (see Chapter 17)

Make a marinade of the dressing ingredients and shake together. Add enough of the marinade to dress the salad, toss again, and refrigerate for an hour. Serve on a bed of Romaine Lettuce with Pimento-stuffed green Olives added.

Serves 4–8.

VEGETABLE SALAD SUPREME

It is really a mistake to give a particular set of ingredients for a vegetable salad because the makings for one of these truly depends on the contents of your refrigerator or your garden. I would hate it if you felt you had to go shopping every time you wanted to make one of my recipes. So please just poke around your house or garden for the herbs, investigate your refrigerator for vegetables, and check out the empty lot next door or search the countryside for some fresh greens. Wash what you've collected, drain it, dry it, tear or cut it into pieces, and put it together in a bowl. Then top with a drizzle of good oil and a squeeze of Lemon juice, toss with a handful of minced herbs, serve it on lovely salad plates, AND eat! One of my recent vegetable salads consisted of:

    diagonally sliced Zucchini
    finely sliced red Cabbage
    diagonally sliced Cucumber
    diagonally sliced Celery

all arranged on a plate. Then I added some sliced Tomato, sprinkled on some Soybean Sprouts, and put on some Avocado slices. I composed the dressing as I went along: a drizzle of Safflower oil, a grand sprinkling of dried Chervil and Fish Herbs (Chapter 17), and then squeezed half a Lemon over all, and added a touch of Tarragon-flavored white wine vinegar (Chapter 17). I looked at the salad and liked it, but then decided to add some Alfalfa Sprouts and some flowers (Nasturtiums and Violets) for color. It was delicious.

FRESH MINT SALAD

Watercress
Romaine Lettuce
Spring Onions
Nasturtium leaves and flowers
Spearmint
Chickweed

Take any assortment and quantity of the greens, wash and drain them, and wrap in a clean terry-cloth towel, and refrigerate. When ready to serve, tear up the greens into bite-size pieces and fill a salad bowl with your assortment.
For a Simple Dressing:
Sprinkle Safflower oil over the greens. This particular salad requires a lighter tasting oil than Olive oil. You could also try Soybean oil. Toss the salad. Just before serving, add salt and Pepper and toss lightly again. Add a tablespoon or two of Tarragon-flavored vinegar or Lemon juice and toss again.

WILD SALAD

Salad:
A salad bowl full of wild greens such as Scallions, Chickweed, young Comfrey, Miner's Lettuce, Watercress, Dandelion shoots, and Nasturtium leaves and flowers.

Dressing:
Mix together 1/2 cup salad oil such as a mixture of Soy-Safflower-Peanut, or Sunflower oil, and 1/4 Lemon juice, 2 T. Honey, a bit of salt and Pepper, and a hint of Garlic.

Wash, drain, and dry the greens. Mix together the dressing and dress the salad with a generous dollop and toss. Decorate the salad with any fresh chopped herbs you have and add some sprouts if you wish.
Serve with Indian Corn Soup and toasted sour-dough French bread for a real old-fashioned meal.

LEMON SALAD DRESSING

Place in a blender and blend together for 2 minutes the following ingredients:

2–3 oz. lemon juice or vinegar
1–2 t. herb salt
4 sprigs Lemon Balm
4 sprigs Lemon Thyme
4 sprigs Parsley
1 sprig Rosemary
1 sprig Marjoram
1 2-inch Lime Geranium
1 2-inch Lemon Geranium

1 leaf Rose Geranium
1 leaf Apple Geranium
1 leaf Nutmeg Geranium
1 small leaf Peppermint Geranium
1 t. dry Mustard
1/2 t. white Pepper
1 T. Lemon honey (any honey will do)
1 T. white wine

Add 4–6 oz. combination vegetable oil* and blend for another minute. Serve as a dressing for marinated vegetables or salad. To make a creamy dressing Yogurt may be substituted for the Lemon juice. To make a dip Sour cream may be substituted for the oil.

*My favorite combination oil is one that includes all the necessary fatty acids, such as equal quantities of Soy, Safflower, Peanut, Corn and Walnut.

Enough for 2 salads.

Chapter 10

Vegetables: Some Green Things for a Luscious Skin

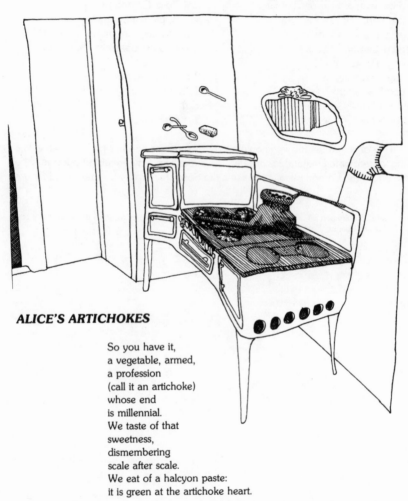

ALICE'S ARTICHOKES

So you have it,
a vegetable, armed,
a profession
(call it an artichoke)
whose end
is millennial.
We taste of that
sweetness,
dismembering
scale after scale.
We eat of a halcyon paste:
it is green at the artichoke heart.

—Pablo Neruda. Reprinted by permission
from the publisher.

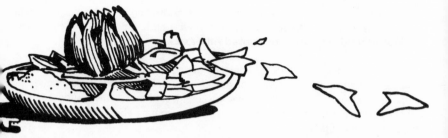

We love the Artichoke in our house and eat it whenever possible in any number of disguises, but we think it most agreeable simply cooked, with a light yogurt and herb dip. Stuffed is fine, Artichoke hearts on an English muffin with a poached egg (Eggs Rosas) is terrific, but for just plain appetizer eating, the simpler the better.

Artichokes	2 stalks Celery with leafy tops
1 Garlic clove per Artichoke	Chicken broth, optional
1 t. Olive oil per Artichoke	1 Onion, chopped
Water	1 Lemon, cut

Cut the stalk off the Artichoke evenly at the base and slice off the upper ¼-inch. If you are particular, evenly cut off the tips of each leaf to get rid of the spiny end. Swoosh the chokes up and down in salted water to get rid of any bugs, and then place them, cut stalk side down, in an enamel pot. Make sure the sides of the chokes touch so that they don't fall over in the boiling water. Put 1 clove of Garlic and 1 t. of Olive oil in the center of each choke and add water to the pot until it recovers the lower two-thirds of the standing chokes. Add the Celery, some chicken broth if you like, and the Onion. Rub the cut surfaces of the chokes with a cut Lemon to prevent discoloration. Bring to a boil and simmer the chokes until tender, about 30–45 minutes or until the leaves can be torn out easily. Remember, leave the top off the pot while cooking to preserve the Artichokes' color and so they won't develop a bitter taste. Take the chokes out of the pot and turn them upside down to drain. Then serve hot or refrigerate until needed.

Artichoke Soup Stock is made with the water the chokes were cooked in. Add a marrow bone and some more vegetables and simmer until all is tender. Then strain out the solid matter and use the liquid as a stock. You could also use the Artichoke water as a liver cleanser "tea" or during fasting diets.

Artichoke Dips can be healthy and easily made if you will only ignore the ubiquitous mayonnaise. Mayonnaise is delicious but much too oily and fattening for most people.

So try various mixtures such as yogurt with Herb Seasoning (Chapter 17); or one-half mayonnaise, one-half yogurt, dash of Lemon juice and Marjoram or Oregano; Hollandaise or vinaigrette sauce on cooked Artichokes.

Artichokes change the taste of wine, rendering it almost sweet, so eat your Artichokes with water, by themselves, or served with a cold, very dry, strong white wine. Some authorities recommended a *vin gris* or Macon, and I have often eaten Artichokes with champagne or zinfandel. Artichokes contain about 2% protein, B vitamins, and some Vitamin C.

ASPARAGUS GREEN GREEN

The Asparagus Green Green makes a delicious breakfast or luncheon dish, and it can be a first course to a fine dinner. It will act medicinally as a diuretic. You can refrigerate the extra sauce and use it later as a salad dressing.

    3 lbs. Asparagus, washed, trimmed,
       and tied in bundles of 6

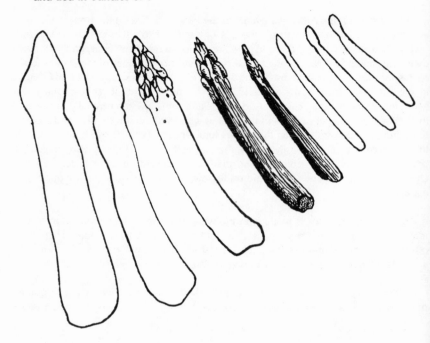

When convenient, or about an hour before needed, boil the tied Asparagus in salted water until it is *al dente*.

Sauce:

2/3 C. vegetable oil
1/3 C. Tarragon vinegar
1/4 t. dry Mustard
2 eggs, hard cooked (chop the whites and sieve the yolks)
3 Shallots, finely chopped

1 Garlic clove, finely chopped
2 T. chopped Capers or Nasturtium buds
1/2 C. fresh chopped Parsley
1/4 C. fresh chopped herbs (Basil, Lemon Balm or Spearmint, Lemon Thyme, Tarragon, etc.)

In a blender combine the oil, vinegar, and mustard and blend for a minute. Then stir in the remaining ingredients. Sample the sauce and adjust the seasonings to your taste, adding a dash of herb salt, if you like. To serve, arrange the Asparagus bundles attractively on a wooden platter. Spoon on a thick layer of your sauce.

Serves 6.

INDIAN CORN

6 C. boiling water
2 C. dried Corn
1 stick (4 oz.) butter
1 yellow Onion, thinly sliced and chopped fine
Maple syrup

1/2 C. cream
1/2 t. salt
Pepper
Corn oil
Paprika or Cayenne
Parsley or Marjoram

Pour the boiling water over the Corn and let it soak overnight. Drain the Corn and reserve the liquid. In a cast-iron skillet melt the butter and sauté the Onion until golden; then add the Corn and stir together. Add 1 cup of the reserved Corn liquid, a bit of Maple syrup, and simmer until the Corn is tender. Continue to add reserved liquid as needed to prevent burning. When the Corn is tender, add the cream and simmer for a few minutes; then add the salt and Pepper and about 1–4 T. of unrefined Corn oil. Transfer to a serving dish, add some Cayenne or Paprika, and sprinkle on some chopped Parsley or Marjoram.

Serves 6–8.

EGGPLANT RATATOUILLE

6 long, skinny vegetables, sliced
   diagonally into 3−4 slices
1 Lemon, juiced
1 t. salt
1 T. Basil, crushed and rubbed
Italian Olive oil

2 Garlic cloves, crushed
1−2 T. butter
1 bunch Spring Onions, sliced
   diagonally
Mushrooms, sliced diagonally
Pepper, freshly ground
1 T. Marjoram

Start with Zucchini or Japanese Eggplant and slice them as directed. Pour the Lemon juice over them, add the salt and Basil, and toss together to combine. Let it rest for a few minutes or refrigerate for a few hours. In an iron skillet add a dollop of Olive oil, the Garlic, and the butter. Cook over low heat, and when the Garlic is soft, add the Onions, Mushrooms, Pepper, and Marjoram, and sauté until slightly tender, about 5 minutes. Remove contents to a holding pan. Drain the Lemon juice from the Eggplant and put the Eggplant in the skillet. Sauté until slightly tender, about 5 minutes. Add more oil as necessary so it doesn't stick. Add the Onion mixture to the Eggplant, give it a light toss, and simmer together until just tender but with a hint of firmness. This dish is best made a day in advance so the flavors can develop. Serve hot, cold, or warm with a crisp green salad and hot millet or rice.

Serves 4−6.

STUFFED MUSHROOMS

This is a very casual dish that is excellent used as a main course for a vegetarian dinner or as an appetizer or hors d'oeuvres at a more elaborate meal. They can be made ahead of time and refrigerated, and then simply warmed up when you need them. Of course, as an appetizer you would probably want to use the little baby mushrooms, and as a main course use the larger ones. But be loose with your ingredients. You can add leftover rice to the mix or even meat.

6−10 large Mushrooms per person
1 Garlic clove, finely chopped, per
   person
Olive oil
Butter
1 Onion, chopped, or a bunch of
   chopped Scallions

1 handful Almonds or assorted Nuts,
   chopped
1 small handful dried Currants
Parsley, minced
Heart's Delight Herbs (Chapter 17)
Dash hot sauce (Bermuda
   Outerbridge's Sherry Pepper
   Sauce)
Hard cheese, grated

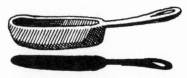

Spoon out or break off the stems of the Mushrooms, leaving a cavity in the cap. Sauté the Mushrooms and Garlic in a mixture of Olive oil and butter until the caps are barely tender. Use a cast-iron skillet for best results. Set them aside to cool in a pie pan or baking pan, capside down, cavity up. Chop the Mushroom stems and mix together with the Onion, Nuts, Currants, Parsley, Herbs, and hot sauce, and put through the coarse grind of a blender or finely chop by hand. Sauté this mixture lightly in the leftover oil and mushroom juices of the same skillet in which the caps were cooked. Let cool. Using a teaspoon, place a small amount of the Mushroom-Nut mixture inside the cap of each Mushroom. Sprinkle each one with grated cheese and set pan in a 350° oven until the cheese is hot and bubbling. Serve garnished with Parsley.

OKRA

"Okra is a Cinderella among vegetables. It lives a lowly life, stewed stickily with tomatoes or lost of identity in a Creole gumbo. . . . I know of no other cook who serves it as I do. To bring it to its glamorous fulfilment, only the very small tender young pods must be used. These are left with the stem end uncut and are cooked exactly seven minutes in rapidly boiling salted water. I serve them arranged like the spokes of a wheel on individual small plates with individual bowls of Hollandaise sauce set in the centres. The Okra is lifted by the stem end as one lifts unhulled strawberries, dipped in the Hollandaise, and eaten much more daintily than is possible with Asparagus. The flavour is unique. The Hollandaise, it goes without saying, must be perfect, just holding its shape, velvety in texture, properly acid. I use the yolk of one egg, the juice of half a lemon, and a quarter of a pound of butter per person."

This recipe is from *Uncommon Vegetables* by Eleanour S. Rohde who found it in Miss Kinnan Rawling's *Cross Creek*.

GARLIC-CHEESE SCALLOPED POTATOES

3 Potatoes, thinly sliced and placed in
    ice water at least 3 hours before
    cooking
3 Garlic cloves, minced
Chicken stock, heated

1 stick (about) butter, thinly sliced
1/2 lb. Swiss cheese (Emmenthaler or
    Gruyère), thinly sliced or grated
1 small Onion, thinly sliced
Salt
Pepper

Drain the Potatoes about 1 hour before needed and dry them on a towel or paper towel. In a casserole make alternate layers of Potatoes, butter, Garlic, Onion, cheese, salt, and pepper. Pour on the heated chicken stock until it just barely covers the Potatoes. Bake in a 375° oven until the Potatoes are tender (30–45 minutes).

Serves 4–6.

SPANAKORISO *(SPINACH AND RICE)*

Contributed by "the Bug" (John Manousos) and his Wife Ann, on the Occasion of their Wedding in which the invited Guests all Contributed to the Feast by Preparing one of the Greek dishes.

To serve 3:	To serve 30:
1 lb. fresh Spinach, washed	10 lbs. fresh Spinach, washed
1 Onion, minced	10 Onions, minced
2 Garlic cloves, minced	10 Garlic cloves, minced
1/2 C. raw brown Rice	5 C. raw brown rice
Olive oil (Greek)	2-1/2 C. Olive oil
1 Tomato	1/2 C. Tomato puree
1/2 Bay leaf	5 Bay leaves
1 C. broth	10 C. broth

Salt and Pepper

Wash and dry the Spinach and tear it into pieces. Sauté the Onions, Garlic, and the Rice in Olive oil until the Onions are soft and golden; add the Tomato and stir together. Add the Spinach, Bay leaf, salt and Pepper, but do not mix. Pour in the broth. Cover and simmer over a low fire for 40 minutes or until the rice is cooked through. This dish is usually served hot as a side dish, but it is also excellent cold.

FAVORITE ZUCCHINI

One year I lived about thirty miles south of Big Sur in an isolated valley of California with nothing to do but look at the gorgeous mountains tumbling into the ocean, and no food to eat but what I grew in the garden. That was the year of Zucchini. Gigantic, luscious specimens grown to perfection on soil treated with water, Camomile blossoms, Nettle tea and compost. The only problem was what to do with all that wholesome food. I made Zucchini salad, stuffed Zucchini, and did everything to a Zucchini that you could possibly imagine. The favorite Zucchini recipe turned out to be this very simple one that my Italian stepmother taught me.

Zucchini   The amount of Zucchini you use depends on the size of the Zucchini. So the easiest thing to do is to take whatever Zucchini you use and slice it crosswise about 1/4-inch thick. If the Zucchini is small, slice it diagonally; if large, cut it lengthwise and then slice it straight across. Slice enough Zucchini to half-fill a skillet.

Bacon   Cut 3−4 strips of bacon into 1-inch pieces and sauté until lightly brown. Drain on newspaper or paper towels to absorb excess fat. Use some of the bacon fat in the skillet to cook the vegetables.

Onion   Slice in thin slices enough sweet yellow Onion to make up half the amount of cut Zucchini. (If you started with 2 cups of Zuke, then use 1 cup of Onions.) Sauté the sliced Onion until translucent in a bit of bacon fat.

Skillet   Layer the sliced Zucchini, cooked bacon, and sautéed Onion in the skillet.

Tomatoes   Squeeze 2 whole, fresh juicy Tomatoes over the top of the ingredients in the skillet. (Don't squeeze with a machine, just take those Tomatoes and scrunch them up in your fist, letting the juice and pulp drop into the pan.)

Seasonings   On top of everything in the skillet, add 1 whole, peeled clove of Garlic (I like three or four, but I am holding back on the amount of Garlic because you may not be ready to use that much), a sprinkling of salt and Pepper, a generous pinch of Marjoram or Oregano, some chopped Basil, and some chopped Parsley.

Cooking   Cover the skillet and steam until the Zucchini is just tender, about 1−20 minutes or until it is done just right for you.

Additions   For variations, heat up this dish with Cayenne or add Parmesan cheese to the top and place under the broiler until the cheese is browned.

Serves 4−8.

AND, believe it or not, this Favorite Zucchini is recommended for people who have acute rhinitis or sinusitis.

There is a wonderful cookbook which gives about 135 recipes using Zucchini, *The Zucchini Cookbook,* by Paula Simmons, published in 1974 by Pacific Search, 715 Harrison Street, Seattle, Washington.

DEBBI'S ZUCCHINI CASSEROLE

1/4 stick (1 oz.) butter
1 small Onion, chopped
2−3 Zucchinis, sliced
2−3 Garlic cloves, minced
Some Basil
3 large Tomatoes, diced and peeled
1/2 lb. cooked chicken, chopped

1 C. Swiss or Mozzarella cheese,
  shredded, *plus* ½ C. for topping
3/4 C. fine breadcrumbs, *plus* 1/4 C.
  for topping
Salt
Pepper
1/4 C. white wine

Melt the butter, add the Onions, Zucchini, and Garlic, and sauté. Add everything else in order of appearance and mix together. Place in a 2-quart buttered casserole. Sprinkle with ½ C. cheese and the ¼ C. breadcrumbs. Bake uncovered in a 375° preheated oven for 30−40 minutes.

Serves 4−6.

Contributed by Deborah A. Putnam, M.D.

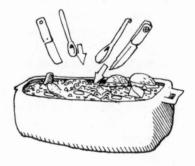

Chapter 11

Beans & Rice, Grains, Maybe Even Bread & Pasta

"He punted back again amongst the waterplants, and took some lunch out of his basket.

" 'I will eat a butterfly sandwich, and wait till the shower is over,' said Mr. Jeremy Fisher. . . ."

—Beatrix Potter, *The Tale of Mr. Jeremy Fisher*

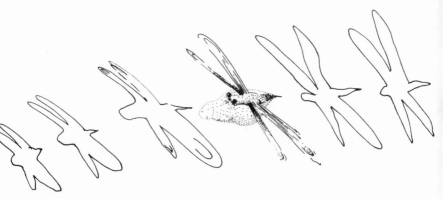

JEAN'S BEANS

We have been baking Beans for decades in our family and have never used any particular quantities. Cooking dried Beans is not as simple as some think. Many factors must be taken into consideration, such as the age of the Bean and the hardness or softness of the water in your area. Cooking time depends on how long you presoaked the Beans and the kind of Bean you are using. It is our custom to use the small white Navy Bean in this recipe, but there are others that will also do.

If you want no-fart Beans, then two things must be done. Soak the Beans for at least 24–36 hours. This starts the sprouting process which breaks down the phytate in the

Bean and allows the zinc in the Beans to be absorbed by the body. Discard the soaking water, water your plants with it, and add fresh water to the beans. Secondly, when you eat the Beans, you must also eat a grass, because a complete protein is formed by the combination of a flower and a grass, such as Beans and Rice, or Corn tortillas and Beans.

Navy Beans	Maple syrup
Water for soaking	Garlic
1/4 lb. smoked or salted pork or salt pork, cut into pieces	Blackstrap molasses
	1/2 t. dry Mustard
1 Onion, sliced	Bean water

Soak about 2 cups of dried Navy Beans in enough water to cover them, plus some; start with about 6 cups of water and add more if necessary. We use bottled spring water that has lots of natural minerals in it. After soaking for 24−36 hours, discard this water and add an equal amount of fresh water, bring the Beans and water to a boil, reduce the heat, and simmer slowly for about 30 minutes. They have cooked long enough when you can take a few Beans into a spoon, blow on them and crack the skin. Foam will rise to the surface as the Beans cook. If it seems dirty, then remove it; if off-white, you can leave it. (I seem to remember something about the foam being composed of a particular amino acid, but simply cannot find the reference nor anyone who can give me the answer.) In any case, when the Bean skins crack, it is time to transfer them to the Bean pot. I sincerely hope that you have a proper ceramic or stoneware bean pot because Beans cannot be properly cooked in anything else.

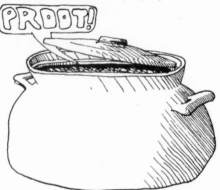

Bean Pot Cooking:
Drain the Beans and reserve the liquid. Grease the pot and put in a piece of smoked pork, an inch or more of the Beans, a slice of Onion, a dollop of Maple syrup, a crushed Garlic, and a tablespoon of blackstrap molasses. Continue this layering until

the bean pot is almost full (pork/Beans/Onion/Maple syrup/1Garlic/molasses). To 1 C. of the reserved Bean liquid add the Mustard and another dollop of Maple syrup and molasses. Add enough of this seasoned liquid to the bean pot so that it just reaches the inside rim. Put on the cover and set the pot in a 250° oven for 5−8 hours or until the Beans are tender. Check the Beans about every hour or so, and if they seem dry, add some of the seasoned Bean water. After 4 hours, if the Beans are not dark enough, add more molasses; if they are too sweet, add a bit of salt and molasses; if they are not sweet enough for your taste, add more Maple syrup. When the Beans are tender, remove from the oven and let rest on top of the stove until cool. Then eat or refrigerate.

These Beans are delicious as a topping on Whole Wheat toast (our flowers and grass idea), or for dinner with whole brown Rice and a delicious green salad. We eat them for breakfast, lunch, or dinner. They are especially tasty the second or even the third day as the flavors develop even more. Don't forget to complete the flower Bean protein with a grass (Rice or Wheat) protein.

Serves 6−8.

HUMMUS BI TAHINI
(GARBANZO BEAN DIP OR SANDWICH SPREAD)

2 C. raw Garbanzo Beans	To serve 50:
2−3 Garlic cloves (I actually like more)	6 C. raw Garbanzo Beans
1/2 t. hot Paprika	6−8 Garlic cloves
Pinch Cayenne Pepper	1-1/2 t. hot Paprika
1/2 C. Tahini (Sesame seed paste)	1/4 t. Cayenne Pepper
1/4 C. Lemon juice	1-1/2 C. Tahini (Sesame seed paste)
	3/4 C. Lemon juice

2 cups of raw Garbanzo Beans will make 6 cups of cooked Beans. Soak the Beans in water overnight, add more water to cover if necessary and bring to a boil. Remove the foam and simmer until tender. Drain the Beans but reserve the liquid, and set aside a small handful of Beans for garnishing. In a blender, Champion juicer, or by mashing with a fork, blend together the remaining ingredients, alternating in adding the Beans, seasonings, and tahini. Bring to a thick, creamy consistency, using the reserved Bean liquid as needed. Adjust the flavor with more Lemon juice and tahini. Add 1 teaspoon of the Seasoning Mixture (see below) (3 t. to serve 50), add more if you like the taste of Cumin, and mix thoroughly.

Put the *Hummus* into a bowl and add the following garnishes. Drizzle on some Greek olive oil. Sprinkle with Paprika. Garnish with chopped Parsley. Top the bowl with the handful of reserved whole, cooked Garbanzo Beans. Serve as a dip with chips or crackers, stuff it in Pita bread with sprouts, or spread on Whole Wheat bread as a sandwich.

Seasoning Mixture:
1 t. salt
1 t. Cumin seed, ground in a mortar
1/2 t. Black Pepper

1/2 t. Turmeric, ground
1/2 t. Coriander seed, ground
2 T. Parsley, dried and minced
1/4 t. Cayenne, ground

This Seasoning Mixture is usually used for Felafel but is delicious in *Hummus,* on eggs, on vegetables, etc.

GARLIC BREAD

1 stick (4 oz.) butter
5 Garlic cloves

1 large loaf sour-dough French bread
1/4 C. good quality Olive oil

Leave the butter to soften in a warm place for a few hours. Put the Garlic through a press and blend with the butter. Add about 1/4 cup of good quality Olive oil (I like Tigres Brand from Italy) to the butter and Garlic, and mash with a fork until it has a paste-like consistency. Slice the bread diagonally two-thirds of the way through. Spread the Garlic butter paste on both sides of each slice of the bread. Wrap the bread in foil leaving the top open to let out moisture, and put into a 350° oven to bake until the top is crisp and the Garlic butter is runny and has oozed into the bread from all sides, about 10–20 minutes. Serve and let your guests tear off as much as they want.

Another delicious way to eat Garlic bread is to go through all the procedures listed above, and then toast it in a dry cast-iron skillet until crisp, and serve as is or with a pasta or fish sauce on top.

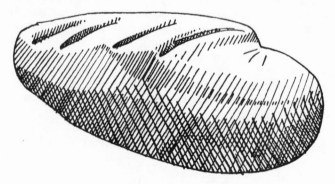

GARLIC CROUTONS

Croutons can be made in exactly the same way as you make Garlic bread. When you remove the bread from the oven, let cool and then cut it up into bite-size pieces. Let the bread cubes dry out before storing in a dry container.

Another method is to take day-old bread, rub each piece on both sides with a cut clove of Garlic, cut up the bread into bite-size pieces, and then toss it with a bit of Olive oil, and store until needed.

Croutons are delicious tossed into your favorite green salad or ground up and used as crumbs in various recipes that call for them, or as the base for stuffing poultry or meat.

BONNIE'S POPOVERS

Popovers are those delicious, bread-like objects that blow up and have a giant emptiness in the center that can be filled with all sorts of good things like tuna or cheese, but we like them filled up with butter and honey. They are delicious. But popovers will only rise if you use all the ingredients at room temperature and use the correct oven temperature. We also feel it is important to use heavy-duty iron popover pans, although other cooks definitely disagree with this idea and hold it is old fashioned.

1 C. all-purpose enriched white, or Whole Wheat pastry flour	1 C. milk
	3 eggs
1/4 t. salt	1 t. sugar, optional
1 T. baking powder (opt.)	1/2 t. herbs, optional

The night before sift the enriched white or Whole Wheat pastry flour (do not use self-rising enriched flour) with a fork. Add the salt and sift again with a fork. Add the baking powder and again sift. (The baking powder is optional according to Bonnie, while I think it is necessary.) Put this into a blender and slowly add the milk while blending at medium speed. Blend for 2 minutes. Add the eggs one at a time, blending each egg into the mixture for 1 minute before adding the next. At this point you may also add the sugar or herbs. The total time for blending will be 5−7 minutes. Set the blender aside until morning. (It need not be refrigerated unless you live in a very hot climate.)

In the morning turn the oven to 425°, butter the popover pans with a pastry brush, and heat them in the oven until they are very warm. (I have found that preheated popover pans are not always necessary to get perfect results.) Blend the popover mixture again for 1 minute. Fill the pans about 1/2 to 2/3 full, put into the oven and bake 30−40 minutes. You may also reduce the heat to 300° for the last 20 minutes if you like. If you wish to freeze the popovers, 10 minutes before they are done, prick each one two or three times with a long, pointed fondue fork to release steam, and then immediately upon removal from the oven pop them into the freezer. When frozen, bag them together in a plastic bag and replace in the freezer until wanted.

Makes 10 popovers.

ORGANIC JOHN'S PASTA PHILOSOPHY WITH ADDED RECIPES

Organic John is a friend as well as a wonderful exciting fanatic on the subject of food. We delight in his ideas and many of his recipes. He has kindly let me excerpt this material from his book, *Let There Be Food* (see Bibliography). This is his way of describing vegetables.

"A walk through Nature's Garden brings on the kind of high that excites the sensory organs . . . The visual richness exclaimed by the silk red of the cherries and the velvety magenta of the eggplants . . . The voluptuousness of the vegetables about to burst, yet so graceful in body. The swaying of the grains while exposing themselves from within their sheaves."

And then John said, . . . "I got so high I made a dish of spaghetti to come down on . . .!"

Use noodles "made with water and the flour of Artichoke, Buckwheat, Spinach, Whole Wheat or Sesame. These noodles do not contain any artificial coloring, preservatives, eggs or honey. Whatever size noodle you choose, served with one of these sauces will become a whole new gourmet experience—light and earthy yet robust and satisfying."

VARIATIONS ON AN AL PESTO THEME

These recipes were adapted from *Let There Be Food* (see Bibliography).
Al Pesto
Blend:

2 bunches of Parsley, chopped
3 bunches of sweet Basil, chopped

Add:

3 cloves of Garlic
1/4 lb. of Pignoli Nuts

1 slice of soya butter
2 oz. Olive oil

Sauté for 3–5 minutes with

1 clove of chopped Garlic
1 oz. Olive oil

You can also add:

2 fresh hand-squeezed Tomatoes

to chopped Garlic and Olive oil.
Cook for 8–10 minutes, then add al pesto.

Variation no. 1
Sauté:

2 cloves of Garlic	1/2 white Onion, chopped
3 Shallots, chopped	2 oz. Olive oil

for 3 minutes. Steam for 3 minutes:

2 bunches of spinach, chopped fine

and add to sautéed Garlic and Onions.

Add:

1 teaspoon cashew butter

and cook for 3 minutes.

Variation no. 2
Blend:

1 lb. Peas

and sauté with

3 cloves of Garlic, chopped	2 Green Onions, chopped
	2 oz. Olive oil

for five minutes.

Variation no. 3
Sauté:

1 lb. of Asparagus

for 5 minutes in

2 oz. boiled water	1 T. mineral powder

Blend with:

2 oz. Olive oil
1 t. Kelp

5 green Olives
3 Mint leaves

Variation no. 4
Steam 1 lb. Fava Beans for 10 minutes in 3 oz. water.
Then blend with:

2 cloves of Garlic
2 oz. Olive oil

10 black Olives
5 raw Mushrooms

FETTUCCINE ALFREDO

1–4 T. butter
1 C. thick fresh cream
Salt

Pepper, freshly grated
Olive oil
1 C. Parmesan cheese, freshly grated
1 lb. fettuccine, fresh

The butter and cream should be at room temperature. Just before you wish to serve the pasta, bring water to a boil and add a bit of salt and a bit of Olive oil. Drop in the fettuccine and cook *al dente*. Drain the pasta, toss it with the butter and the cream and half of the cheese. Grate fresh Pepper over the top of the fettuccine, and pass the pasta with the rest of the cheese around the table.

Serves 4–8.

Chapter 12

Meat (Meat, Poultry, Fish and Seafood)

"And instead of a nice dish of minnows—they had a roasted grasshopper with lady-bird sauce; which frogs consider a beautiful treat; but *I* think it must have been nasty!"

—Beatrix Potter, *The Tale of Mr. Jeremy Fisher*

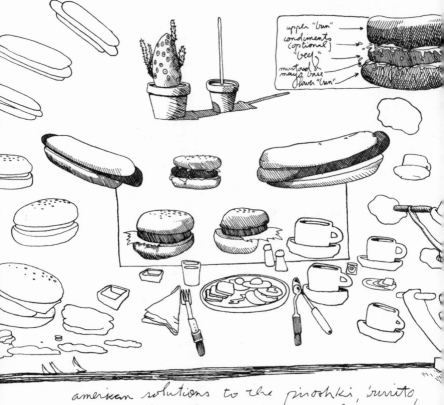

american solutions to the piroshki, burrito, wonton, Kuo Teh, and/or dumpling (meat)

A GOOD OLE COUNTRY HAM

Before I moved to northern Florida with a south Georgia family, my idea of a ham was the watery, pudgy pink stuff that people covered with cloves and brown sugar and served, sliced at crummy cocktail parties. As a matter of fact, I believe they were called "party hams." These squooshy pieces of meat always made me slightly sick to my stomach. But then I moved to Florida, and one memorable Christmas my south Georgia friend took me shopping for a HAM. We cruised around several butcher shops where hams, salted, smoked, lean and thin, hung. Some were rolled in black pepper, some were growing blue mold. They were all very interesting and looked rather repulsive, but I was assured that the taste would more than compensate for their present looks. And it certainly did. I like ham now and eat it occasionally. In Chapter 6, listed under Virginia and Tennessee you will find the addresses of several good ole country ham makers who sell their goods by mail-order.

First, find a good salt-cured and smoked ham. Scrub it thoroughly and soak it in cold water for at least 24 hours to remove some of the salt. Put the ham in a large pot and cover it completely with water. Add a good-sized handful of brown sugar to the water. Let it come to a boil, and then reduce the heat and simmer the ham for 20–25 minutes per pound. Keep the ham covered with water. The ham is done when you can pull out the end bones easily. Cool the ham in the pot in its own liquor. When it has cooled enough to handle, take it from the pot and remove the skin. Score the fat, dot it with cloves and sprinkle with brown sugar. Put the ham in a shallow pan in the oven and bake it at 400° until it is brown. Cool and slice it thinly.

I have found that it takes about 6 hours to boil the ham. So if you want a thinly sliced ham for a special occasion, think ahead. You may have to start the boiling process the day before or at 4 or 5 A.M. in order to have it ready for a late afternoon holiday meal.

Serves 10–20.

INDIAN STEW WITH LAMB

Salt
Pepper
Small handful of Spearmint
1 T. Oregano, fresh if possible
6 Juniper berries, crushed with the back of a knife
3–6 cloves Garlic, crushed with the back of a knife and peeled

Corn oil
2 big yellow Onions, peeled, thickly sliced and chopped
1 hot red Chile, crushed
1 C. dried Corn that has been soaked for 24 hours (or 1 large can hominy)
water

1/4 C. Whole Wheat flour
2 lb. lamb, cut into 1 inch cubes

4 green or red Bell Peppers, washed
   and quartered
1/2 C. chopped fresh Parsley

Add the salt, Pepper, Spearmint, Oregano, Juniper berries, and Garlic to the flour. Dredge the lamb with the seasoned flour and brown slowly on all sides in a heavy iron Dutch oven. Remove the meat to a holding dish, add a bit more oil to the pot, and sauté the Onions, Chile and Garlic. Return the meat to the pot. Add the soaked Corn and enough water to just cover the contents. Simmer for 2 hours. Keep checking the pot and add water as needed. Add the Bell Peppers and simmer until tender. Add the Parsley and set the pot aside while you set the table and make a salad; then serve.

Serves 4–6.

LAMB STEW IN A PUMPKIN

1 Pumpkin, approximately 8–10
   inches in diameter
2 lbs. good, tender lamb stew meat
1/4 C. Whole Wheat flour
1 t. salt
1/4 t. fresh Pepper
1/8 t. Cinnamon, ground

1/8 t. Ginger, ground
Bit of ground Lemon Peel
Olive oil
1 Onion, sliced
1 Bell Pepper, cut into pieces
1 Carrot, cut into 1-inch pieces
1 C. hot broth

Get a good sized Pumpkin and cut off the top about one-fourth of the way down. Clean the pumpkin out, saving the seeds to be toasted later. Cut out most of the Pumpkin flesh and cube it, but leave about a half-inch thick shell. Toss the lamb meat in a paper bag to which you have already added the flour, salt, Pepper, Cinnamon, Ginger, and Lemon Peel. Heat Olive oil in a cast-iron skillet and brown the flour-seasoned meat. Add the Onions, Bell Pepper, Carrot, and Pumpkin cubes to the skillet, and cook until slightly soft. Put the vegetables and meat into the hollowed out Pumpkin shell. Add 1 cup of hot broth. Cover the Pumpkin with its lid. Put it into a baking dish with about 1 inch of hot water in the bottom of the dish. Set the oven at 350° and bake until the Pumpkin is tender. Add some cooked Peas and some sliced Pimentos to the Pumpkin stew and serve it.

Serves 6–8.

ARROZ CON POLLO
(CHICKEN WITH RICE OR RICE WITH CHICKEN)

1 chicken, organically grown and fed, or a kosher chicken
1/2 C. Spanish Olive oil
2–4 Garlic cloves (two, if your children don't like Garlic)
1 Spanish yellow Onion, sliced
1 t. Oregano, rubbed between the palms

1 t. Sage in leaf form, rubbed between the palms
1 T. Saffron or more
2 chiles, hot and small, optional
1-1/2 C. water or chicken broth
1 C. short or long grain whole rice
2 Tomatoes, thinly sliced
1 large handful of Mushrooms, sliced
1 green Bell Pepper, thinly sliced
butter
1 can whole Pimentos, thickly sliced

Wash the Chicken in cold water, pat it dry with a muslin towel, and cut it up any way you like. Brown the chicken, Garlic, and Onion in Olive oil. Use an old-fashioned cast-iron Dutch oven, as cooking in these pots will give you over a period of time quite a bit of absorbable iron. Because our culture is lacking in this substance, it would be a good idea to make it a habit to use cast-iron ware more often. Now, if for some reason you have purchased a supermarket chicken, it will be more watery and less chicken-juicy than one organically grown. You will have to reduce the amount of oil in which the chicken is browned.

When all the chicken parts are nicely brown, remove the beast and the Onions from the oil with a slotted spoon to a holding dish. Add the Oregano, Sage, Saffron, and Chiles to the oil and juices in the Dutch oven and sauté for a few minutes. Then add the water, Rice, and Tomatoes. When this comes to a boil, return the chicken and Onions to the pot. Simmer over a low flame for 20 minutes. Remove from the heat. Let the flavors blend and marry for about 6 hours. Sauté the Mushrooms and Bell Pepper in a bit of butter. Add to the top of the Arroz con Pollo, with the Pimentos. Reheat over a low flame for 20 minutes or until hot. Serve from the Dutch oven.

Serves 4–8.

Menu Suggestion:
Arroz con Pollo
Large green salad, tossed with Oil and Lemon
Bold red wine
Fruit for dessert

GARLIC CHICKEN

20—40 garlic cloves
1/4 C. Olive oil

1 stick (4 oz.) butter
1 plump roasting chicken, organically
grown

Mash the Garlic with mortar and pestle, or press through a Garlic press. Mix the Garlic with the Olive oil and butter. Wash and dry off the chicken, and salt the inside and outside by putting a tablespoon of salt in your hands and thoroughly fondling the chicken. With your fingers gently loosen the skin from the flesh, especially around the breast and thighs. Cover the flesh of the chicken (under the skin) with the garlic mash by pushing it in all the cracks and crevices of the chicken with your fingers. (Just grab some of the garlic mash and push it under the skin and around the breast and thighs). Cover as much of the flesh as you can reach. Pull the skin back over the body of the bird. Put it in a roasting pan in a 375° oven and roast until done.

Serve this delicious chicken with a fresh, crisp salad, whole grain rice, and a glass of red wine.

Serves 3—6.

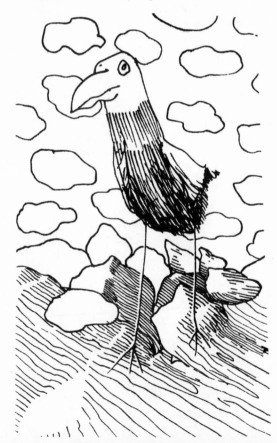

STEAK TARTARE

1 lb. ground steak
1 handful minced Parsley
1/2 Lemon, juiced
2–4 Garlic cloves, pressed
1 egg yolk, beaten frothy
1/4 C. minced Onion (or more)
1 t. Dijon-type Mustard, hot
1 T. drained Capers or pickled
  Nasturtium seedpods
1 T. anchovies, freshly chopped

Seasonings:
  All or some, to your taste
  1 T. Olive oil
1 t. Worcestershire sauce or
  Outerbridge's Sherry-Pepper sauce
Salt
Freshly ground Pepper
Dash of hot sauce (like Tabasco) or
  red oil (Chapter 17)

Get the very best quality steak (use lean meat and cuts known as eye round, top sirloin, or top round) and have it ground to order. Then proceed to mix everything together. Shape this into a nice round mound, refrigerate until chilled, and serve as an hors d'oeuvre with a robust red wine and crackers. A good food if you are protein deficient and carnivorous by nature.

STEAK TARTARE #2

1 lb. ground round
4 T. mayonnaise
1 T. chopped Parsley
2 sweet pickles, minced
4 anchovies, chopped

1 t. chopped Capers
1 t. dry Mustard
1 Garlic clove, minced
Worcestershire sauce
Dash Tabasco
1 small chopped or grated Onion

Mix all together.

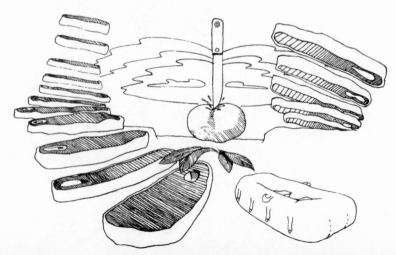

CHILE COLORADO

Every so often I get the mad desire to eat something so hot, so Chile-red hot, that I have to go to my favorite Mexican restaurant here in San Francisco, Roosevelt Tamale Parlor, and order Chile Colorado. This madness strikes me about three times a year and off we go; the children order Beans and Rice, Mike orders *Flautas,* and I eat the heat. I think that it puts a disordered digestion back together and opens the blood circulation system so that it can operate more coherently. For me, it cheers me up and heightens my sense of perception. I have experimented with many recipes, and I think I like this one best.

1 lb. tasty beef, cut into bite-size pieces	1 t. Oregano
2–5 Garlic cloves, crushed	Dried Cumin seeds
1 C. hearty red burdgundy	Chicken broth
4—8 hot red Chiles	1 T. Whole Wheat flour
	Corn oil
	Salt to taste

Sauté the meat and Garlic in some Corn oil in a heavy cast-iron skillet or Dutch oven until brown. Add the wine to the meat and start simmering. Remove the stems and as many of the seeds from the Chiles as you like (the seeds are extremely hot and somewhat bitter and add or subtract to the taste of the finished dish, depending on the quantity you use), and parch them separately in a heavy skillet for a bit. Turn off the heat and add a little bit of chicken broth, water, or wine to the Chiles to soften them. Then use a mortar and pestle to mash the Chiles, Cumin, Oregano, and a bit of salt until pasty. Add the chicken broth until you do have a paste. Brown the flour in 1 T. Corn oil and gradually add the Chile-paste mixture. Slowly stir this into the meat and simmer, covered, for about 1 hour or until the meat is tender. You can eat it right away served over rice, or you can cool and refrigerate the "hot" meat to let it age a day or two before reheating to eat.

If you happen to get any of the Chile oil under your fingernails or in your eyes, remember that the best first aid remedy that you have available is plain Yogurt. You can apply the Yogurt generously anywhere on your body, including in the eyes. Also, Yogurt makes a great cool-down food while you are eating this fiery delicious dish.

Serves 4–6.

HOLIDAY TURKEY

Recently it has been my honor and pleasure to be the official cook of our Christmas turkeys at the family get-togethers. I like using a nice organically grown (fed naturally, no hormones, etc.) turkey. I make a mixture of butter, Olive oil, crushed Garlic, lots of rubbed sage, dash of Cinnamon, dab of Cloves and a pinch of Cumin. This mixture is then spread smoothly over the turkey flesh but under the skin. I loosen the skin from the body by inserting my fingers between the skin and the flesh. It seems as if the turkey can almost be totally removed from the skin. Then the turkey is stuffed (see Turkey Stuffing recipe), sewn up, and put on a rack breast side up in a large baking pan. A clean muslin dish towel or cloth is then dipped in water, wrung out, and laid over the turkey, tucking the ends in around the legs. We cook it at 300° for about 20 minutes to the pound (20 min./lb. for a bird under 15 lbs., and 15 min./lb. for a larger bird). The cloth-wrapped bird *MUST* be basted with a brush every 15 minutes in the beginning and then every 30 minutes as juice collects. The basting juice is either the drippings in the bottom of the pan or else a blend of melted butter and oil. Just brush the muslin cloth as often as it needs so that it doesn't dry up. (Do not remove the cloth to baste, but baste the cloth instead.) DO NOT put foil under the bird as this will stick to the cooking beast leaving a mess for you to clean up. When the bird is done, remove from the oven and let it rest for 30 minutes to an hour before it is carved. I can guarantee you that this will be one of the most delicious divine foods that you have ever tasted.

TURKEY STUFFING

1 stick (4 oz.) butter
2 Onions, chopped
4 stalks Celery, finely sliced
2–8 whole Garlic cloves
2 sweet Red Bell Peppers, chopped
Peanut oil
1 C. coarsely chopped or sliced
 Mushrooms

2 T. mixed seasonings (like the
 poultry seasoning in Chapter 17)
1 C. chopped nuts (Peanuts and
 Cashews)
1 C. chopped Parsley
½ C. Wheat germ
1/2 to 1-1/2 lbs. Whole Wheat
 croutons (depending on size of
 turkey — 8 oz. of croutons equals
 about 6 cups)
Salt, Soy sauce, brandy, optional

Sauté in the butter the Onions, Celery, Garlic, and Bell Peppers. In a larger pan, sauté the mushrooms in Peanut oil. Combine the contents of the two pans and add the mixed seasonings, nuts, Parsley, Wheat germ, croutons. Add salt if you like, and maybe some Soy sauce or brandy. Give it a few good stirs with a large wooden spoon. Lightly spoon the stuffing into the cavity of the turkey.

Makes 10–20 cups.

TURKEY STUFFING FOR THE NECK

Turkey giblets, finely chopped
Butter
1 bunch Spring Onions, finely
  chopped
1 qt. oysters, drained and chopped
Celery, finely chopped

Parsley, finely chopped
1 Garlic clove, crushed
Dash of Cayenne Pepper
Lavender Buds
Tarragon
Cooked whole Rice or wild Rice

visp

Sauté the giblets in butter and add the Spring Onions. Sauté until almost done. Add the oysters and sauté for a bit longer until married. Add a bit of Celery, Parsley, the Garlic, Cayenne, and maybe some Lavender buds or Tarragon, and, if you have it, some cooked whole Rice or wild Rice. Combine all ingredients and stuff the neck cavity.

Makes 2–4 cups.

BOUILLABAISE (A FISHY STEW)

1 yellow Onion, coarsely chopped
  and sautéed in some olive oil
3 juicy Tomatoes, coarsely chopped
5–10 cloves of Garlic, chopped
the green tops of Celery, chopped
1/2 bunch Parsley
1 sprig fresh Fennel
1 stalk fresh Thyme
1 piece broken Bay leaf
2 pieces Orange peel

Tie together in a cheesecloth bag or
use an equivalent amount of dried
herbs; for example, 1 T. Parsley, 1/2 t.
Fennel, and 1/4 t. Thyme.

1/2 lb. Clams
1/2 lb. Lobster or Crayfish
1/2 lb. Prawns or Shrimp
1/2 lb. or more Oysters on the
  half-shell
other assorted shellfish, like Mussels
  and even Crabs
2 lb. assorted fresh fish, like halibut,
  sea Bass, red snapper
up to 1 cup good Spanish olive oil
salt and freshly ground or crushed
  Black Pepper
a few Cloves
1 t. Saffron (more if desired)
1 qt. white wine
1–2 qt. water

Put all the ingredients up to the sea foods in a large, deep soup kettle. Pour on some of the Olive oil and cook for a few minutes. On top of this scented garden of delights add some of the Saffron and the shell fish in layers. Cut the fish into large pieces and alternate the various fish on top of the shell fish. Pour over this the rest of the Olive oil, the salt and Pepper, the Cloves, some more Saffron if you like, and enough white wine and water to just cover the fish. Bring to a bubbling boil and immediately lower the heat and simmer only long enough to properly cook the fish, about 15 minutes.

To Serve:

Rub Garlic over slices of dry sour-dough French bread and put a nice slice in each deep soup plate. Separate the soup stock from the seafood. Put the stock into another hot serving bowl and ladle it over the bread in each bowl. The fish and shell fish are served separately, arranged in a large, deep round dish standing on another dish. Tuck slices of fresh French bread around the edges of the lower dish. Each diner takes what he or she likes of the seafoods, adding some vegetables from the bottom of the soup kettle to the seafood or soup as they desire.

Please try to remember that a bouillabaise recipe is really only a suggestion. You must use whatever seafood or shellfish is in season. It is probably best to stick to what is freshly caught, and if you live in California, what could be more delicious to add to your soup than some crab in its shell or even some freshly pounded abalone. We have also made the bouillabaise with freshly sauteed Mushrooms as an addition. Please, please do not overcook this dish, as there is nothing so soggy and unpleasant to eat as overcooked fish that tastes like mush. We also like to add a red or green Chile pepper or two for added zip, and even squeeze Lemon juice into the soup plate. Garlic is nature's most fantastic antiseptic and will clean your liver as it enlivens your intestines. I really like using the red Italian Garlic in my bouillabaise, but as that is not always available, use whatever you've got.

You might make *aioli* and serve it along with the toast. Whenever I make this soup I think of Palo Colorado Canyon and Bidwell, and having dinner with him in his snug cabin under the gorgeous redwoods with a giant fire burning fragrantly in the fireplace.

Serves 8.

CHINESE-STYLE STEAMED FISH

4–5 lb. Red Snapper or other firm, white-fleshed fish

Azuki beans, salted

1/8 C. Chinese rice wine

1 Onion, sliced

1/8 C. toasted Sesame oil

1/4 C. good quality Soy sauce

1 piece fresh Ginger

2 Garlic cloves, crushed

Szechuan Peppercorns, crushed

1 red Chile, optional

4 Spring Onions with tops, sliced diagonally

Fresh Cilantro (Coriander tops, Chinese Parsley)

Clean the fish, leaving the head on. Wash the fish thoroughly inside and out and dry it. Rub the inside of the fish with salted Azuki beans. Mix together the wine, Onion, Sesame oil, Soy sauce, Ginger, Garlic, Szechuan Peppercorns, and the Chile. Pour this mixture over the fish and soak it for several hours.

Use a pan with a rack to hold the fish at least one inch off the bottom of the pan. Put the fish in the pan, belly side down with the sides opened out. Pour over it the soaking mixture. Cover the pan and steam it over medium heat for about 20−40 minutes until almost done. Meanwhile diagonally slice the Spring Onions and tear up some fresh Cilantro. Put half of this mixture over the fish and steam for 15 more minutes, or until done. To test, insert a fork and the flesh will flake when done. Place the fish on an attractive serving platter with the rest of the Onion and Cilantro decoratively covering the top. Add more Soy sauce and crushed Garlic if you wish.

Serves 8.

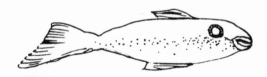

BALM-WRAPPED FISH

1 T. vegetable oil
1 whole fish or fish steaks (2−3 lbs.)
3 Garlic cloves, crushed
Salt (Lemon salt would be nice here)
Pepper

10−15 long Lemon Balm sprigs
1−2 thickly sliced sweet yellow
   Onions (Maui Onions, if possible)
Some white Grapes
Some white wine

Put a bit of vegetable oil in a baking pan. Rub your fish with the Garlic, some salt and Pepper. Wrap the fish in the Lemon Balm sprigs, and put them in the pan. Cover the fish with the sliced Onions (to add flavor and to hold the sprigs in place). Sprinkle some Grapes over the top. Add enough wine to get a little liquid in the bottom of the pan, probably no more than 1/4−1/2 cup will be needed. Cover the pan and place in a moderate 350° oven for 30−40 minutes or until the fish is cooked.

When we use this recipe we do it with different kinds of fish. Red Snapper has a great texture but often Halibut tastes better. You could try several different kinds of white-fleshed fish.

Serves 2−4.

STEAMED FISH WITH DILL

2 T. Olive oil
1 large sweet yellow Onion, thinly sliced
4 peeled Garlic cloves
1 bunch Dill weed with seed

3−5 lb. whole fish or piece of fish (Halibut is perfect)
soft butter
Garlic
white wine (Muscat type is good)

Cover the bottom of a heavy cast-iron Dutch oven with Olive oil, and sauté the Onion and Garlic until they are almost tender. Remove them from the pan and lay in the Dill weed. Rub the fish with the butter and a bit of Garlic. Put the fish, belly down, on the Dill weed bed and fold the Dill over the top. Cover with the Onions and the Garlic. Pour in the wine. Cover the pan and steam until the fish is done, about 20 minutes per lb.

Serves 3−6.

LIME-DILL LING COD (OR OTHER WHITE FISH) FILLETS

3 lbs. fish
2 Limes, juiced
1/3 C. dry Sherry
1 C. cold water
1 C. white wine
6−8 Cloves
1 Onion, chopped fine

2 Carrots, chopped fine
1 stalk Celery with leaves
Parsley sprigs
1 T. Dill seed
Paprika
Alfalfa Sprouts, Watercress, or other edible greens

Marinate each side of fish in a mixture of Lime juice and dry Sherry in the refrigerator for 1 hour. Starting with the cold water and wine, simmer the remaining ingredients to make a broth. Drain the marinade from the fish and place the fish in a lightly oiled baking dish. Use Safflower oil. Strain the broth and pour over the fish. Add enough broth to almost but not quite cover it. Place in the lower third of a preheated 350° oven, and poach from 12−20 minutes depending on the size and thickness of fish. Do not overcook.

Make your favorite sauce with the leftover stock from baking, or serve cold in a gelatin glaze and layer according to the rule for gelatin. Sprinkle with Paprika. Garnish with Alfalfa Sprouts, Cress, or whatever edible green you wish.

Serves 3−4.

Contributed by Eve Travis.

Chapter 13

Other Eggs, Quiche, Fondue

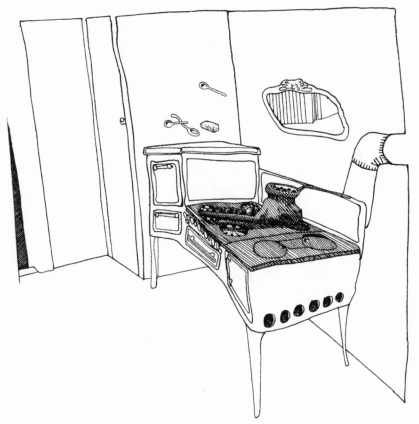

"Generally, all cheese unsalted, that is to say, fresh and greene, is good for the stomach. Old cheese stoppeth a laske,* abates flesh and makes the body lean . . . The cheese made of goats milk, stamped into a cataplas and so applied, healeth the carbuncles engendred about the private parts"

Pliny's Natural History,
28th Book

*diarrhea

AMBER'S FAVORITE FONDUE RECIPE

Fondue does not have to be a tricky thing to make. We have found that if you will just start with the best ingredients, (as with anything), you will come out with a superb product.

1 lb. Gruyère cheese, or 1/2 lb. Swiss and 1/2 lb. Gruyère, or 1/2 lb. Gruyère and 1/2 lb. Caraway cheese
Whole Wheat flour
1/2 t. Fines Herbes (Chapter 17)

1 – 2 loaves extra sour-dough French bread
2 C. white wine (Riesling, Chablis, or Champagne)
1 T. Lemon juice
1/4 C. Kirsch
Nutmeg, freshly ground
White Pepper
Cayenne

In the morning, dice the cheese into ½-inch cubes and dredge with a small handful Whole Wheat flour that has had the Fines Herbes added. Set aside in a bowl, but do not refrigerate. (There are countless varieties of cheese; Gruyère is saltier than most and more strongly flavored than the preferred Emmenthaler or Swiss cheese.)

Cut the loaves of sour-dough French bread into pieces about 1-inch square, leaving a piece of crust on each. Set aside in a bowl to dry out, or start with stale bread.

To Cook and Serve:

First give your guests a delicious, crisp green salad, pour yourself a glass of wine, and start making your fondue. We use a classic earthenware fondue pot *(caquelon)* and prefer it to any other for making a really delicious fondue. But you can use any flameproof pot if it can stand direct heat.

Rub the fondue pot and a large wooden spoon generously with a cut clove of Garlic. Pour into the pot 2 cups of a dry white wine (Champagne, Riesling, or Chablis), any wine acid enough to melt the cheese. Place over a moderate heat. When small bubbles start to rise to the surface, add the Lemon juice.

Add the cheese to the pot, one small handful at a time, constantly stirring it in a figure-eight movement with a wooden spoon. I have also used an egg beater, but this is strictly a no-no for most cooks. Wait until each handful is melted before adding another. Stir until the mixture is lightly bubbling. Transfer to the warming plate on the table, and finish your fondue with a flourish.

Add the Kirsch or other brandy, a dash of Nutmeg, a grind of white Pepper, and a sprinkle of Cayenne. Continue to stir with the wooden spoon in a figure-eight pattern to keep smooth. Each guest spears a piece of bread with a fondue fork, dips it into the fondue, and eats a piece of heaven. Serve with chilled white wine.

Serves 4 – 6.

Editor's note: If a person loses the bread on their fork, the penalty is for them to drink the remaining wine or beer in their glass before they are permitted to dip into the fondue again.

THE FIRST QUICHE

I am a lousy pie crust maker so when making quiche I usually choose to do one of two things. Buy a ready-made pie crust from the grocery store, which is usually inferior to one I could make. Or ask friend Penny to make a pie crust for me!

1 9- or 10-inch pie crust, baked with 1/2 T. Fines Herbes added to the dough

6–10 slices of bacon; crisply cooked and cut into 1-inch pieces, or sautéed Mushrooms

1 Onion, thinly sliced and sautéed until golden in a bit of bacon fat

1 C. grated Gruyère cheese, or extra sharp Cheddar

4–5 eggs

1-1/2 C. creamy milk or half-and-half

Sesame salt

White Pepper

Pinch Nutmeg

Butter and Parsley to garnish

Preheat the oven to 375°. To the baked pie crust add, in layers, the crisply cooked bacon (or the Mushrooms), the sautéed Onion, and the grated cheese. Beat together the eggs, milk, and seasonings until well blended. Place the pan on the bottom rack of the oven, and pour in the egg mixture. Leave room at the top of the crust for the eggs and cheese to puff. Dot the top of the quiche with bits of sweet butter. Slide the rack back into position and bake about 30 minutes or until the quiche puffs, is brown, and a toothpick inserted in the center comes out clean. Garnish with Parsley.

Serves 4–6.

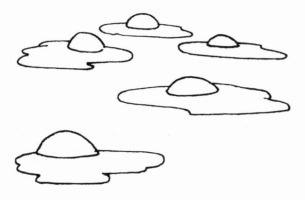

THE BRIE QUICHE

1 9-inch deep dish pie crust
4 eggs, beaten frothy
1 1/2 C. creamy milk or half-and-half
1/2 t. Cumin, or seasoning
mixture from Hummus bi Tahini

Sesame salt
White Pepper
1 Onion, thinly sliced and sautéed in
  a bit of butter
4–6 oz. Brie, sliced thinly

Mix together the eggs, milk, and seasonings, and beat with a wire whisk. Pour half of this mixture into the pie crust, and add the Onions. Layer on top half of the thinly sliced Brie. Pour over the top the rest of the egg mixture and then add evenly the rest of the Brie. Bake in a preheated 350° oven until a fork can be inserted and removed cleanly, about 30–40 minutes. The Brie melts deliciously inside the egg mixture while it gets crispy and brown on top. Truly a delicious combination.

Serves 4–6.

Editor's note: I was lucky enough to be in San Francisco, working with Jeanne on this book, the day she made this *terrific* quiche. After many hours of laboring together, Jeanne disappeared into the kitchen and returned with this yummy snack. "Jeanne," I said, "you must add the recipe to your book." And so she has—you'll love it too!

Chapter 14

Snacks & Hors D'Oeuvres

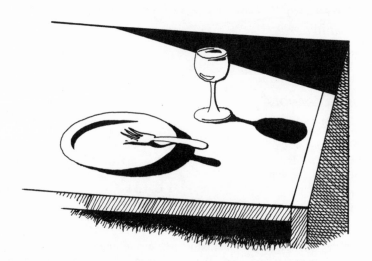

PENNY'S ALL STAR GRANOLA

The best granola is one that is very fresh.

2−4 C. Oatmeal
2 C. finely shredded coconut
2 C. Wheat germ
4 C. or more of coarsely chopped
dried fruits and nuts such as Dates,
Bananas, Apricots, Almonds,
Cashews
Rye flakes, optional

Bran, optional
Soybeans, toasted, optional
Seeds, optional
Cinnamon, ground, optional
1/3 C. oil, such as Peanut, Corn, or
Safflower
2/3 C. Maple syrup
1 t. Vanilla
1/3 C. warm water

Combine in a shallow pan or on a cookie sheet the Oatmeal, coconut, Wheat germ, and dried fruits and nuts. Mix these ingredients well with the hands and spread out evenly on the pan or cookie sheet. You may also add to your taste Rye flakes, Bran,

Soybeans, Seeds, and Cinnamon. Mix together the oil, Maple syrup, Vanilla, and water, and pour over the dried mixture. Place the sheet in a preheated 350° oven and bake 15 minutes. Use a spatula to turn over the mixture and continue to bake 15 minutes longer. After baking the granola, allow it to cool on the cookie sheet. It will have crunchy lumps for good snacking. Store at room temperature in an airtight container or cannister. In cooler climates granola need not be refrigerated.

Makes about 10 cups.

Courtesy of Penelope Hallinan.

GRAMMY'S GRANOLA

6 C. rolled Oats	1/2 C. honey
1 C. Sunflower seeds	1/4 C. butter
1 C. Sesame seeds	1/4 C. molasses
1 C. shredded coconut	1/4 C. water
2 t. salt	1 C. raisins
1 T. Cinnamon	1 C. Wheat germ
	1 C. chopped nuts

Mix together the Oats, seeds, coconut, salt, and Cinnamon. Heat together the honey, butter, molasses, and water. When well blended, pour over the dry mixture and mix it well. Spread it on two cookie sheets. Bake in a preheated 300° oven for 15 minutes. To each cookie sheet add 1½ cups of the mixed raisins, Wheat germ, and nuts. Bake again for 10 minutes. Stir again. Turn off the oven heat but leave the sheets in the oven another 10 minutes or until cool. Store in large-lidded containers in the refrigerator. Serve with milk or yogurt, or fruit juice and yogurt, or eat dry as a snack.

Makes about 10 cups.

Courtesy of Sally Moore (Mrs. Bryan S. Moore)

CORN CHIP SNACK

Corn chips	Sweet Onion, thinly sliced
Sharp Cheddar cheese, grated	Guacamole

In a baking pan alternate layers of Corn chips, grated cheese, and thin slices of sweet Onion. Bake in a preheated 350° oven until the cheese has melted. Serve with a large dollop of guacamole on the top.

To eat, pull out a cheesy Corn chip from the mound and dip in the guacamole. It is really delicious. Potato chips can be substituted for the Corn chips.

OLLIE'S ONIONS

Water enough to cover the Onions
1 lb. sweet Onions (such as Maui Onions), unpeeled
{ 1 C. dry white wine
{ 1 C. water of the reserved Onion water
   Or
2 C. dry white wine
2 T. honey
2 T. Olive oil
6 Juniper berries, crushed

1 Lemon, juiced
Sesame salt
White Pepper
1 small Bay leaf
Some Lemon Balm (may be to lemony)
1 T. white wine vinegar
1 T. Olive oil
3 Juniper berries
Parsley, chopped
Thyme or Tarragon

Bring the water to a boil, add the Onions, and boil them for a minute to loosen the skins. Remove the Onions, top, tail, peel, and slice them thinly. To one cup of the reserved water in the pot add the Onions along with the remaining ingredients, except the wine vinegar, Olive oil, and 3 Juniper berries. Simmer the mixture until the Onions are just tender. Remove the Onions with a slotted spoon to a holding dish. Boil up the remaining liquid in the pot until it has thickened. Pour over the Onions and chill in the refrigerator overnight. Drain and pour the juice into a stock pot. Add to the Onions the wine vinegar, Olive oil, and 3 Juniper berries. Toss and chill. Sprinkle with chopped Parsley, Thyme, or Tarragon before serving.

Serves 4–6.

Chapter 15

The Sauce

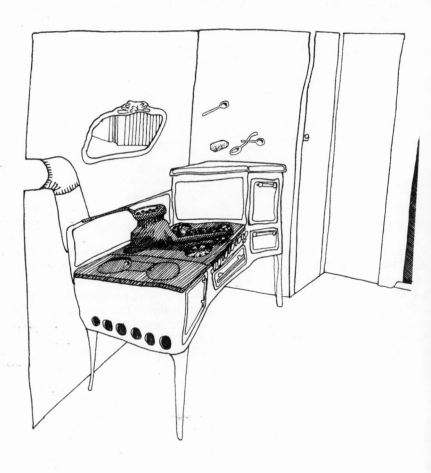

RED CHILE SAUCE
(SALSA COLORADO)

12 red Chiles, heat will depend on the
    type and hotness of your red Chiles
2–5 Garlic cloves, sliced
3–6 Tomatoes, peeled and halved
1 sweet red Bell Pepper
1 C. claret, chicken broth, or water

2 T. Corn oil
1 T. Oregano
1/2 t. Cumin seed
1/4 t. Thyme
1 T. red wine vinegar or apple cider
    vinegar
Salt to taste

Deseed and destem the Chiles, and then parch them in a cast-iron skillet. Add the Garlic and sauté for a minute. Add the Tomatoes and the red Bell Pepper, the liquid, and simmer for a few minutes. Remove to a blender and blend until coarse. Or, better yet, beat it or grind it by hand with a mortar and pestle. Meanwhile, add the oil to the skillet along with the rest of the spices, and sauté until the fragrance begins to be released. Add the vinegar and the blended Chile mixture. Salt to taste. Heat and simmer until the flavors have married. This is delicious over Beans and Rice, or as a sauce for enchiladas or meat. It can be hot or sweet, depending on the type of red Chiles you use.

Makes 2–4 cups.

YELLOW CHILE SAUCE

4 yellow Chiles
2 yellow Crookneck Squash
1 yellow Onion
Cilantro, crushed

1–5 Garlic cloves
1/2 C. Chicken broth
Salt
Tahini
1 Mexican Lime

Deseed and destem the Chiles and coarsely chop them and the Crookneck Squash, and slice the Onion. Put them in a blender with the crushed Cilantro, Garlic cloves, and the chicken broth. Whirl it briefly. Add salt to taste, and tahini if you would like to gentle the taste. Remove mixture from the blender, and add in the juice of the Lime. Mix with a spoon. Hot and delicious.

If your Chiles are very hot ones, this can be *HOT*. You can control the heat of this sauce by the type and number of Chiles that you use, as well as the amount of tahini you use to gentle the sauce. I like to eat this over eggs and in some Mexican foods. It will last in your refrigerator up to two weeks, so freeze some if you do not think you can eat it all in that time.

Makes 2 cups.

A GOOD GARLIC SAUCE FOR VEGETABLES
(ALSO FOR FISH OR USED AS A DIP)

2 large Potatoes, boiled, then peeled and mashed with a fork
6–10 Garlic cloves, pressed or crushed

1/2–1 C. good Olive oil (the type of Olive oil determines the taste—I prefer a Spanish Olive oil here
1/3–1/2 C. Lemon juice, freshly squeezed, or herb-flavored wine vinegar
Salt
White Pepper
Herbs (Tarragon is good)

Mash the Garlic and Potatoes together with a fork until smooth. While mashing, slowly alternate adding the oil and Lemon. Add 2 parts of oil to every 1 part of Lemon juice. Add the seasonings and whip until everything is thoroughly mixed. Now taste the saucy dip and alter the seasonings or thin with Lemon juice, Olive oil, or chicken broth. There are many vegetable and nut variations of this good Garlic sauce, any of which should be ground to a paste in a mortar or blended and added during the Garlic-Potato mash. These variations include: Almonds, tahini, honey, Avocado, cooked Eggplant, or cooked Carrots.

Serves 4–6.

YOGURT-GARLIC SAUCE

1–4 Garlic cloves
Salt or powdered Kelp
1/2 C. Yogurt
Goodly pinch of herb, rubbed between the palms, (herb depends on what the sauce is for)

Some Suggested Combinations:
Mint with lamb
Dill or Fennel with Fish
Basil with Tomatoes or over cottage cheese
Chives or Parsley with eggs
Sage, Lemon, or Tarragon for Chicken

Finely chop the Garlic and then pound it with a pestle in a mortar. Add the salt and pound to a paste, while slowly adding the Yogurt. When it is really smooth, taste the mix and add more salt if necessary. Stir in the herb.

Besides the uses mentioned above, this Yogurt-Garlic sauce is excellent to eat by itself for disordered digestion, and it can be applied to insect bites or some skin irritations.

Makes 2/3 cup.

GUACAMOLE

Several large Hass Avocadoes (the ones that are really oily, tasty, and with a thick skin)
Lemon juice
2 green Chiles, or 1 hot green or red Chile, fresh or canned, deseeded and destemmed, if necessary, and chopped
Salt
Pepper
2 Garlic cloves, crushed
Dash Cumin
2 large Tomatoes, coarsely chopped
1 bunch Spring Onions, finely sliced
Cilantro

Peel, remove pits, and mash the Avocadoes with a fork. Add the Lemon juice, Chiles, salt, Pepper, Garlic, and Cumin. Combine the chopped Tomatoes and sliced Onions and add to the mix. Adjust the seasoning to your taste. Put into a serving dish and sprinkle Cilantro over the top.

Serves 4−6.

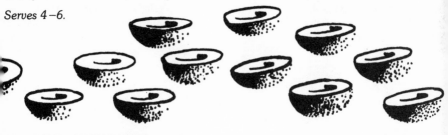

BLENDER MAYONNAISE

Oil for
an olla's
epiphany,
the partridge's pedestal,
keys to a mayonnaise heaven.

—Pablo Neruda/217.
Reprinted by permission from the publisher.

1 egg
1/4 t. Mustard, dry
1/4 t. salt
1/2 t. sugar (optional)
pinch of Cayenne or Garlic or Parsley (optional)
4 t. acid (Lemon juice or Apple cider vinegar)
4−6 oz. good vegetable oil

The trick to mayonnaise is blending in each ingredient slowly. By the end of the beating the blender heats up slightly and seems to aid in the emulsifying effect by its slight cooking action. So drop the egg in the blender and run it on medium speed for 3 minutes, add sugar and blend 1 minute, and add any optional ingredients and the acid and blend for 1 minute. You have now had your blender going for 7 minutes and now is the time to start adding the oil *drop by drop* off the end of a teaspoon. As the mixture starts to thicken, the oil can be added in larger amounts. The addition of the oil should take about 10 minutes. Towards the end of the blending time the mayonnaise will begin to emulsify and firm up. From time to time stop the blender and push the mayonnaise, using a flexible spatula, down from the sides and onto the blades.

I have made mayonnaise with all kinds of oil from unrefined Olive and Soy to the highly refined commercial products. Naturally, the more flavorsome the oil the more flavorful the mayonnaise. My husband likes a rather bland but tasty mayonnaise made with refined but non-heat-treated Soy and Safflower oil, while I prefer the rich full taste of this spread when made with Italian Olive oil. In any case, you can make all sorts of dressings with this mayonnaise. For example, add Garlic mashed to a paste in a mortar and pestle, or add large handfuls of chopped Parsley or Basil for a green dressing, or blend in some Avocado for a Green Goddess style of salad dressing. This mayonnaise is good with sandwiches, salads, stuffed Avocadoes, and as a cleansing cosmetic for the complexion.

Makes 1 cup.

PESTO SAUCE FOR BREAD AND NOODLES

1 C. fresh Basil leaves
1/2 C. fresh Parsley, finely chopped
1/4 C. Pine nuts
2–4 Garlic cloves

Olive oil, enough to moisten, start with 1/4 C.
1/2 C. or more Parmesan cheese
Salt to taste
Pepper to taste

Chop the Basil and combine it with the Pine nuts, Garlic, Olive oil, and half the Parmesan in a blender. Blend just a few seconds. Stop the blender, push down the herbs. Add more oil and cheese if desired, and blend a few more seconds. Salt and Pepper to taste. Serve with freshly prepared pasta. We like the tagliarini verde. Cook the pasta al dente, and toss it with a bit of butter and Olive oil. Put the pasta in a serving dish and cover with the Pesto sauce. Toss and serve. Pass around extra Parmesan or Romano cheese.

Serves 4–6.

PARSLEY SAUCE FOR BREAD, VEGETABLES, OR NOODLES

Use the above recipe. Simply substitute Parsley for Basil. Small amounts of other chopped herbs can also be added, such as bits of fresh Thyme, Oregano.

SHIRLEY'S SALSA MEXICANA

This delicious sauce always accompanies meals in Mexico. It is served over breakfast eggs, seafood, steaks and other meats. Tacos are improvised with tortillas, fresh or fried, bits of chicken, cheese or any leftover meat and *Salsa Mexicana*. It is thought to cleanse the digestive system, ridding the intestines of parasites and amoebas—those troublesome ailments referred to as "Montezuma's Revenge."

2 C. chopped fresh Tomatoes
  (skinned, if you prefer)
3/4 C. chopped Onion

2 T. chopped hot green Chile
  Peppers
1 T. chopped Cilantro
1 t. salt
Juice of 2 Limes

Combine all ingredients and refrigerate before serving to allow the flavors to blend.

Courtesy of Shirley Boccaccio.

SALSA VERDE #1
(GREEN SAUCE)

5 medium-hot green Chiles
2 hot green Chiles
3 fat Garlic cloves
1 green Bell Pepper
1 Zucchini
1/2 bunch Spring Onions

Parsley or Watercress (Parsley is
  cooling, Watercress is hotter)
Raw Corn oil
1 handful Pumpkin seeds
1 T. Coriander seeds, whole
1 sprig Epasote
1 t. Cumin seed, whole
1 C. water with 1–2 T. Soy sauce
  added

Deseed and destem the Chiles, and slice the Chiles and Garlic into thin slices. Cut the green Bell Pepper into eighths and then cut crosswise into half-inch segments. Quarter the Zucchini lengthwise and slice thinly. Slice the Spring Onions diagonally, and chop the Parsley or Watercress. Keep all these vegetables in separate little piles. Put a couple of tablespoons of Corn oil in a cast-iron skillet, and heat until hot. Add the Pumpkin seeds and toast until they start to pop. Then add the seasonings and the vegetables, one at a time, starting from the top of the list. As you add each vegetable, stir it around a little before adding the next one. When everything is mixed together, and while the vegies are still crisp, add the water and boil away until about half of the water is gone. Simmer for a few more minutes, turn off the heat, and cover. Cool and store in a jar, or eat right away. We find this delicious hot sauce great as a topping on a poached egg, over rice, or served separately as a side dish. It is also good eaten as is for a sore throat. Try it, you'll like it.

Makes about 2 cups.

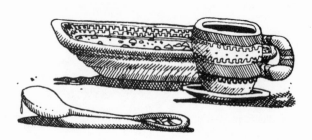

SALSA VERDE #2
(KNOCK YOUR SOCKS OFF HOT SAUCE)

6 long green Chiles (mildly hot)
4–8 short green Chiles (hot)
1/4 C. Sunflower seeds
1 C. chicken broth
2 Garlic cloves

1/2 Onion, chopped
1/4 C. Corn oil
1/2 bunch Parsley, chopped
Celery tops, chopped
Salt to taste

Deseed and destem the Chiles. Sauté the Sunflower seeds in a bit of the oil and put them in the blender with the Chiles. Blend until coarse and add the chicken broth. Sauté the sliced Garlic and the Onion in the rest of the Corn oil, and add the contents of the blender. Heat gently. Add the Parsley and the Celery tops and heat briefly. Salt to taste, and bottle with a tight-fitting top to age for a day or two before using. This sauce will last in the refrigerator for up to two weeks. It can also be frozen for later use. Regulate the heat of the sauce by the proportion of long green to short green Chiles you use.

Makes 2 cups.

Chapter 16

Desserts — Those Yummy Things You Don't Need to Eat

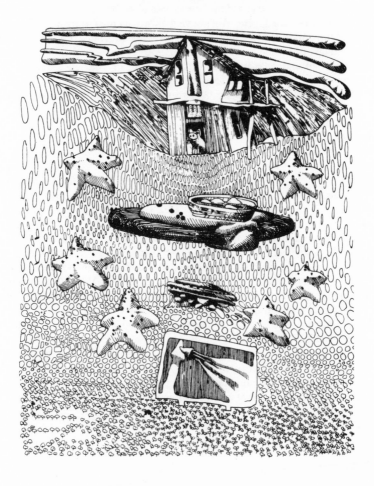

BRYAN'S POUND CAKE

My best recipes are accidents, mostly someone else's accident. Take this morning, for instance. Bryan, age two, got up early but soon came into the bedroom laughing gleefully about eggs. Stumbling into the kitchen, I found a dozen eggs cracked on the table and onto the rug, with a few having managed to sneak their way into the bowl—with the shells, of course. Well, having always wanted to make a pound cake, this seemed the opportune moment. The problem was, how to extract the shells from the bowl and also remove a pound of partially ground Coffee beans the dear boy had also dropped into and onto the eggs. First, I got out my kitchen scale, put on it a 2-quart bowl to weigh, and started to add the eggs that were broken on the table. The eggs with the shells and the Coffee beans I strained through a colander with small holes. And from here you can begin your recipe.

- 1 lb. eggs (1 dozen)
- 1 lb. sweet butter
- 1 lb. sweet (brown sugar or Maple syrup)
- 1/2 t. Vanilla oil, or 1 t. Vanilla extract
- 1/2 t. ground mace
- 1 T. Rosewater or Orange flower water
- 1 lb. Whole Wheat flour, sifted
- 1/2 t. cream of tartar, optional
- 1/2 t. salt, optional

Add eggs into a large bowl until they weigh one pound, and beat them with a mixer until frothy. In a separate bowl cream the butter and slowly stir in the brown sugar or Maple syrup. Cream the butter and the sweet you've chosen, and slowly blend in the frothy eggs, a little at a time. Beat the batter very well. Add the Vanilla (oil is better than extract*), the mace, and the Rosewater or Orange-flower water. Sift the flour and to it add, if you like, the cream of tartar and the salt. Add the flour mixture to the egg-butter-sugar mixture. Mix together and beat for 100 strokes. Pour into a greased loaf pan and bake at 325° for 45–60 minutes. Of course, my procedure differed somewhat as I started out with egg shells and Coffee beans (some of the ground beans had gotten into my mix and I discovered that they were good for added flavor).

In any case, the result is a dense, tasty cake that is best eaten in thin slices with tea or Coffee. It can be frozen for future use. Do you wonder what I did with all those Coffee beans? They were washed and placed in the oven, alongside the pound cake, dried, rebagged, and used for Coffee later on in the week.

Makes 4 pounds.

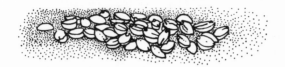

DEBBI'S CHEESECAKE

Now that you are all healthy from using the previous recipes in this book and you are dying for an incredible sweet—Try this!

1 C. graham cracker crumbs
1/2 C. Vanilla wafer crumbs
2 T. sugar
1-1/2 t. ground Cinnamon
2 T. finely chopped Macadamia nuts
6 T. melted butter
8 oz. cream cheese

1/3 C. sugar or 1/4 C. mild honey
1 egg
1/4 t. Vanilla
1 C. sour cream
1 T. sugar
1/4 t. Vanilla
1 C. fresh Raspberries, Blueberries, or cut-up Strawberries

To make the crust, mix together the cracker crumbs, wafer crumbs, 2 T. of sugar, the Cinnamon, nuts, and melted butter. Pat the mixture into a 9-inch pie pan. (The crust proportions vary according to the whim of the cook.)

To make the filling, beat together the cream cheese, sugar or honey, egg, and 1/4 t. Vanilla. Pour into the pie shell and bake in a preheated 350° oven for 20 minutes, or until set. Remove from the oven and turn up the thermostat to 500°. Meanwhile, mix together the sour cream, 1 T. sugar, and 1/4 t. Vanilla to make the topping. Add the topping and the fruit to the cheesecake and bake at 500° for 5 minutes. Cool the cake and chill in the refrigerator before serving.

Serves 4–6.

Contributed by Deborah Putnam, M.D.

*Available from Indiana Botanic, see Chapter 6.

THE BEST DARK FRUITCAKE

2–3 lbs. nut meats (Almonds,
  Pecans, Walnuts, Cashews)
8 lbs. fruit (Citron, Lemon peel,
  Orange peel, Lime peel, honeyed
  Pineapple, home candied Cherries,
  Raisins or Currants, honeyed Figs,
  pitted Dates), one-half should be
  Raisins or Currants
1/2 C. Apricot brandy
4 t. ground Cinnamon
1/2 t. ground Allspice
1 whole Nutmeg, grated

1/2 t. ground cloves
1 lb. dark brown sugar, or 1 lb.
  cooking Maple syrup
1 C. dark molasses
1 lb. butter
1 lb. Whole Wheat pastry flour
10 egg yolks, beaten until foamy
10 egg whites
1/2 t. Salt
Whole Almonds, whole candied
  Cherries, whole candied fruits and
  nuts for decoration
Jamaican rum, optional

Coarsely chop the fruits and nuts and combine. Mix together the brandy and the spices, and pour over the mixed nuts and fruits. Work together until creamy the sugar or Maple syrup, molasses, and butter. Beat the flour and egg yolks into the creamed mixture. Beat the egg whites and salt until stiff, then fold them into the creamed mixture. Pour this batter over the fruit and nuts, and combine these two mixtures. You may have to work them together with your hands. The dough should be stiff and not runny. If it is runny, add more nuts and flour. Grease your pans, (old fruitcake pans work well), and line them with heavy wax paper or parchment paper. Grease them again. Fill the pans three-quarters full. Decorate the cakes artistically with whole Almonds, whole candied Cherries, and whole candied fruits and nuts, such as Apricots and Pecans. Place in a 300° oven for 3–4 hours, or until firm. Place a pan of hot water on the bottom of the oven to keep the cakes moist, but remove the pan of water during the last hour of baking. Remove the cakes from pans and cool on racks. Splash some Jamaican rum or more brandy, about 1 T. to 1/4 C., on each cake. When the cakes are cold, strip off the paper and wrap each one in clean brandy-soaked cheesecloth. Put them back in their pans (very useful are old fruitcake pans with lids), and cover. Store in a cool place but do not refrigerate.

Aging is very important to develop the flavor, and it can be the really hard part of fruitcake making. A fruitcake should age at least one month before being eaten, and ideally three months. The cake has to be opened weekly and good quality alcohol added to it to keep it moist and to preserve it. I prefer using a combination of dark rum and good brandy, and use 1–2 tablespoons of this mixture drizzled over each cake at these weekly intervals. Eventually, when the cake has been soaked enough to seem moist and be fragrant, (four drizzles worth or four elapsed weeks), I wrap it up and let it rest until eating time.

Eating is the last part of fruitcake making. These cakes are very rich and tasty and should be very thinly sliced, each slice to be totally savored and enjoyed before being eaten. They taste especially good with coffee and can be a nutritionally satisfying and relaxing way to start or end the day.

Makes 15 pounds.

When Penny and I last made fruitcake, we scoured the neighborhood for really good quality candied fruits. Some of it was impossible to find. So do look for the best quality fruits *before* you make your cakes, and don't wait until the last minute and maybe have to make do with second-rate fruits. We used what was available at the time, and that is what I suggest you do. Look around, get the best, and don't settle for that diced-up candied junk that you get at the local supermarket.

Last Christmas, my dark fruitcakes were made with the following amounts and kinds of fruits and nuts:

1 lb. Almonds	1/4 lb. candied cherries (natural, not artifically colored)
1/2 lb. Pecans	1/4 lb. Spanish orange peel (dried, from the herb shop, soaked in honey and water until soft)
1/2 lb. Cashews	
1/2 lb. Walnuts	
1 lb. Dates	1/4 lb. candied Pineapple
3 lbs. Currants	1/4 lb. candied Papaya
1 lb. Figs	1/2 lb. Citrons
1/2 lb. Honeyed Apricots	Dried Pears
	Candied Lemon peel
	Candied Angelica stems

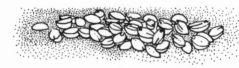

PERSIMMON DELIGHT

1 1/4 C. sugar	1/2 t. Nutmeg
1-1/2 C. all-purpose flour	3 eggs
1 t. baking soda	1/2 C. melted butter
1 t. baking powder	2-1/2 C. whole milk
2 t. ground Cinnamon	1 qt. Persimmons
1 t. ground Ginger	1 C. Raisins

Mix the dry ingredients together and sift into a large bowl. In a separate bowl mix the wet ingredients together. Combine the dry and the wet ingredients, and stir in the cut up Persimmons and the Raisins. Spoon the batter into a well-greased 9x9-inch cake pan, and bake in a preheated slow 325° oven for 1 hour, or until firm.

Serves 4–6.

Contributed by Marshall Krause.

SAVOY'S BIRTHDAY CAKE

Savoy is the daughter of a friend, who is eight or so years old, and who presented this cake to her mother. It's a gooey treat and the last one in this chapter. I think it fitting that a two-year old should have made the first dessert in this chapter and another child the last.

Make a basic chocolate cake recipe, adding chocolate chips and chopped bananas. Let it cool in the pan and then turn it out on a serving plate. The melted chips create their own frosting. Savoy frosted her cake for effect, and for flavor contrast, with her mother's favorite cream cheese frosting.

Frosting #1:

Beat cream cheese with honey and sour cream to a spreadable consistency. (This frosting is also delicious on carrot cake.)

Frosting #2:

Whip cream cheese with grated Orange rind and Orange juice to a nice spreadable consistency. This is terrific as frosting on a cake topped with Mandarin Orange segments arranged in a flower-like pattern.

This particular mixture can be used as a delicious alternative to the usual sugary, tooth-decaying, attitude-changing sweet. Use it as a filling, a frosting, or a spread.

Serves 6–8.

Chapter 17

Other Herby Things: Herbal Blends, Beverages, Jellies & Butters, Vinegars & Mustards, Honeys & Candies

Cottontail and Peter folded up the pocket-handkerchief, and old Mrs. Rabbit strung up the onions and hung them from the kitchen ceiling, with the bunches of herbs and the rabbit-tobacco.

—Beatrix Potter, *The Tale of Benjamin Bunny*

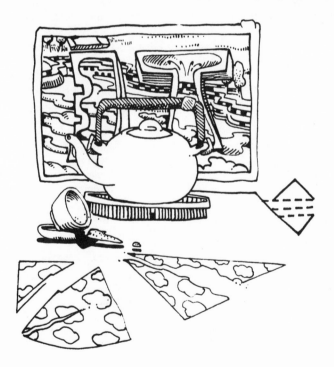

HERBAL BLENDS
(FOR VARIOUS PURPOSES)

When using dry herbs from a store, select good quality ones with strong color and taste. Rub the herbs together between the palms of your hands to remove any large stems and then hand chop them coarsely, or rub them with your hands until they are in fine particles but not powder. Mix together your different herbs and then store in lightproof containers, ideally in a cool, dark place. When starting with fresh herbs, the procedure is the same, except that first you pick and carefully dry the herbs.

All-Purpose Herb Blend
1 part each of:
  Basil
  Bay leaf (1 only)
  Marjoram
  Parsley
  Sage
  Thyme

All-Purpose Herb Blend
THE SALT SUBSTITUTE
1 part each of
  Basil
  Celery tops or Lovage
  Curry powder
  Dulse
  Parsley
  Tarragon
To 1/2 part each of:
  Horseradish
  Lemon Peel
  Oregano
  Pepper, Green
  Rose Hips
  Sage
  Thyme

Bouquet Garni
tie together for easy removal later
  Bay leaf, 1 only
  Marjoram, 1 sprig
  Orange rind, 1 piece
  Parsley, 1 sprig
  Thyme, 1 small sprig

Delicious Delight
(Also a salt substitute)
1 part each:
  Basil
  Chervil
  Lovage
  Oregano
  Parsley
  Rosemary
  Savory
  Tarragon
  Thyme

Fine Herbes
1 part each:
  Chervil
  Chives
  Parsley
  Tarragon

Fish Blend

1 part each:
   Basil
   Dill Weed
   Fennel Weed
   Lavender (1/2)
   Lemon Balm
   Rosemary

Meat Blend

1 part each:
   Bay leaf (1/2)
   Garlic Tops
   Marjoram
   Parsley
   Rosemary
   Thyme

Poultry Blend

1 part each:
   Celery tops or Lovage
   Chervil
   Marjoram
   Parsley
   Sage
   Savory
   Thyme (1/2 part only)

Salad Blend

1 part each:
   Basil
   Celery tops or seed
   Chervil
   Dill Weed
   Lemon Balm
   Marjoram
   Parsley

Soup Blend

¼ cup of each:
   Basil
   Bay leaf (2 leaves crumbled)
   Celery tops
   Marigold petals
   Oregano
   Parsley
   Sage
   Savory
   Thyme (⅛ cup only)

Spaghetti Sauce Seasoning

1 part each:
   Garlic tops
   Marjoram
   Oregano
   Parsley
   Rosemary
   Sage
   Savory
   Thyme

Vegetable Blend

1 part each of:
   Celery
   Chervil
   Dill Weed (1/2)
   Fennel leaves
   Lemon Balm (or Lemon Peel)
   Lovage
   Paprika
   Parsley
   Tarragon

*Note: Meadowbrook Herb Garden, Wyoming, Rhode Island, has a fine collection of well-grown, nicely blended herbal combinations if you prefer to buy rather than to make your own.

CURRY: There are *many* types of Curry powder mixtures. Curries vary considerably, from season to season and even within the same country as well as from different geographical locations. Try this mixture, but also try others.

Curry Powder Blend
4 oz. crushed Coriander seed
2 oz. ground Turmeric
1 1/2 oz. ground Cumin
1 oz. ground Fenugreek seed
1/2 oz. ground Black Pepper
1/2 oz. ground Poppy seed
1/2 oz. ground Ginger powder
1/2 oz. ground Chiles
1/4 oz. ground Mustard seed
1/8 oz. ground Cardamon seed

Curry Powder Ingredients
May contain four-or-more of:

Allspice	Cumin
Almond	Fenugreek
Anise Seed	Garlic
Asafoetida	Ginger Root
Black Pepper	Ginger Tops
Cardamom	Mace
Chiles	Mustard Seed
Cinnamon	Nutmeg
Cloves	Poppy Seed
Coconut	Turmeric
Coriander	

HERB SALTS

Herb salts can be used at the table as a condiment to flavour foods or for cooking. They are extremely useful for people who must reduce the amount of salt (sodium chloride) they consume. There are herbs that have a rather "salty" taste, and there are herbs that provide vitamins and minerals other than sodium.

The blend called All-Purpose Herb Blend, given earlier in the chapter, can be used as a salt substitute where a limited intake of sodium is desired, while the blend called Delicious Delight eliminates sodium altogether.

Other herbal salts can be made by using equal quantities of Bay salt and dried, ground up herbs. Also, some herbs such as Mint for Pea soup or lamb chops, or Basil for Tomatoes can be used.

Basil Salt:
Dry and rub finely 2 T. of Basil. In a small seed grinder, grind 4 T. of Bay (or regular or sea) salt with 2 T. of Basil. Bottle it.

Sesame Salt:
Toast 4 T. of Sesame seeds lightly in a dry cast-iron skillet. Add them to 2 T. of salt and lightly grind together in a small seed mill. This salt is a delicious condiment and once you start using it, you will discard your plain old salt shaker forever.

Spiced Salt:

Blend together the following until fine: 2 oz. salt, 1 oz. Lovage, ½ Savory, ½ Marjoram, pinch of Cayenne or hot Paprika, pinch of Cloves, pinch of Nutmeg, 1 heaping tablespoon Sage, and a largish pinch of Cinnamon. Bottle and use it freely on meat, vegetables, or fish.

Garlic/Onion Salt:

Grind together in a mortar and pestle until fine: 1 T. dried Garlic tops, 1 T. Onion flakes, 1 T. dried Parsley, 1 t. dried Lemon Balm, 1 t. dried Basil, 1 t. dried Chervil. Then grind in 2—6 T. of salt. Bottle for use.

HERB BEVERAGES

HERB TEAS are made for drinking pleasure by bringing a pot of water to a brisk boil and pouring this water over the fresh or dried leaves or flowers of the plant you wish to savor. The quantities are usually 1 pinch or 1 teaspoon of the plant to 1 cup of water, and they should be infused (steeped) for 3 minutes. If you wish a more medicinal drink, use a larger quantity of the plant and infuse longer (1 oz. herb/2 cups water/20 minutes). Naturally, some mild tasting herbs require more in the cup to give a really good flavor. Lemon Balm and Spearmint are two of these. Try loosely filling a pot with either of these fresh herbs and then pouring on the boiling water. I also like to add a bit of honey to the pot rather than to the cup when making herbal teas as the herbal liquid then remains attractively clear. Any herb can be made into tea. The favorites are: Linden, Spearmint, Hibiscus, Camomile, and Lemon Balm.

HERB WINES can be made in two separate ways: 1) actually making wine with the blossoms, or 2) simply infusing flowers or herbs in grape wine already made.

DANDELION WINE

For every quart of the freshly picked blossoms allow:

1 qt. water	Juice and rind of 1 Orange
A little Ginger root	1 T. yeast for winemaking
2 Cloves	2 lb. loaf sugar

Boil all the ingredients, except the yeast and sugar, for 1 hour. Strain, add the sugar and boil it up again for 30 minutes. When nearly cool, add the yeast and mix it thoroughly. Put it into a stone crock container and let it work for two weeks. Skim off and discard foam. Pour into bottles and cork. Age for six months.

BIRCH WINE and Birch Syrup *(Betula alba)* are made from the young leaves that have been picked in the spring, when the growth and the life forces are at their peak. This has a cleansing effect and Birch wine is often used as a spring tonic for people over 35 whose metabolism is changing and possibly slowing down.

ELDER BLOSSOM WINE

Nine pounds of white sugar, three gallons of water, two teaspoonfuls of Lemon juice, one yeast cake and one quart of Elder blossoms picked from the stems.

Boil the sugar and water together, take off while boiling hot, and stir in the flowers. Do not boil these. When cool, add Lemon juice and yeast, put all together in a stone jar, and stir every day for nine days. Then strain through a cloth, chop in three pounds of raisins, and put into the cask. In six months it will be ready to use. (This is a family recipe and very good.)

　　—Katherine van de Veer, *(Herbs for Urbans—and Suburbans)* 1938

CARNATION PINK WINE

To every bottle of white wine, infuse as many pinks as you happen to have. One-half cup of flowers to a quart of wine would be about right, but using one cup of pinks will work also. Let the flowers infuse for several hours before serving. (Straining is not necessary.) This wine is thought to be useful to restore all the body senses.

LEMON BALM WINE

To every bottle of white wine (a mild German wine is preferred), infuse 1 large handful of freshly picked, clean lemon balm. Infuse for several hours before serving. This wine is used to revive sagging spirits.

ROSEMARY WINE OR LEMONADE

Infuse 1 heaping T. of fresh Rosemary tops in a bottle of white wine or freshly made Lemonade. Leave the Rosemary in the wine at least 3 days and in the Lemonade at least 3 hours. (Straining is not necessary.) Rosemary is used for affections of the head and to improve the memory.

ANGELICA LIQUEUR for digestion

Chop, very small, 1 oz. of fresh Angelica stems (before the plant flowers), and steep them in 3 cups of brandy or cognac for 5–10 days. Strain through a fine strainer (muslin or a silk cloth will do). Make a supersaturated sugar-water mixture by boiling water gently and adding sugar to it until the sugar will no longer dissolve. Cool this sugar-water and add about 1 cup or more of it to the Angelica liqueur. Add a drop or two of essence of bitter Almond.

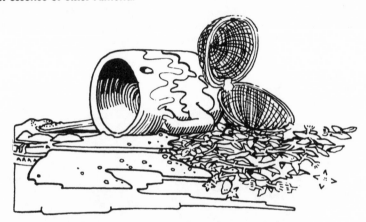

SEVERAL SORTS OF MEATH, SMALL AND STRONG (MEAD)

Small. Take ten Gallons of water, and five quarts of honey, with a little Rosemary, more Sweetbryar, some Balme, Burnet, Cloves, less Ginger, Limon Peel. Tun* it with a little barm;* let it remain a week in the barrel with a beg of Elder flowers; then bottle it.

Very strong. Take ten gallons of water, and four of Honey. Boil nothing in it. Barrel it when cold, without yest. Hang in it a bag with Cloves. Elder-flowers, a little Ginger and Limon Peel; which throw away, when it hath done working, and stop it close. You may make also strong and small by putting into it Orris-roots; or with Rose-mary, Betony, Eyebright and Wood-sorrel; or adding to it the tops of Hypericon with the flowers of it; Sweet-bryar, Lilly of the Valley.

*tun is a type of barrel and barm is the yeast formed during fermentation of alcoholic beverages.

APPLE DRINK WITH SUGAR, HONEY, &c

A very pleasant drink is mad of Apples, thus: Boil sliced Apples in water, to make the water strong of Apples, as when you make to drink it for coolness and pleasure. Sweeten it with Sugar to your tast, such a quantity of sliced Apples, as would make so much water strong enough of Apples; and then bottle it up close for three or four months. There will come a thick mother at the top, which being taken off, all the rest will be very clear, and quick and pleasant to the taste, beyond any Cider. It will be the better to most taste, if you put a very little Rosemary into the liquor, when you boil it, and a little Limon-peel into each bottle, when you bottle it up.

—the Closet of Sir Kenelm Digbie Knight Opened, 1669

MARIGOLD WINE

Making wine from marigolds seemed so preposterous that I had to select a deep orange variety to get at least a redish wine color. Blind faith and the lack of anything else to make country wine drove me to pick the profusion of marigold flowers that I had planted as companions to my vegetable plants. Companionship is now incidental as the marigolds are carefully tended to make one of the most charming and marvel-ously intoxicating wines in my cellar. When the marigold hedges are in full bloom, during August and September on the East Coast, they are picked by snapping them with a satisfying plop between thumb and forefinger at the point where the calyx narrows to the stem. Plastic bags filled with flowers can be dropped into a freezer if your schedule is too full to make wine in the peak of the harvest season.

Flowers are thin gruel when it comes to feeding yeasts. They are generous with fragrance, bouquet and intoxicating properties, but offer little in the way of real nutrition for the yeast. Orange juice and grapefruit juice, frozen or freshly squeezed, with the proper amount of sugar or honey and some malt syrup makes a must that ferments rapidly and can have flowers added to it once a brisk ferment is in progress. The procedure is to get together well scrubbed utensils that have been subjected to boiling water. A stainless steel or non-metallic container of sufficient capacity for the batch of wine contemplated (usually the bigger the better), a stirring spoon, and good lid are all that is needed. Obsessive cleanliness is important because there are thousands of microscopic creatures who would like to eat the delicious must that you have created and only one type will make it into wine, which can be bread yeast, but if at all possible it should be a wine yeast, available by mail-order or in the wine supplies stores.

The Recipe (in gallons which can and should be scaled up)

One gallon of good water	1 C. + orange or grapefruit juice or 1
No more than 2½ lbs. sugar or 3 lbs.	C. lemon juice (freshly squeezed is
honey	best, but frozen will do)
	1 T. malt syrup (optional, but the
	yeast likes it)
	10 to 12 oz. marigold flowers

Boil the water and when it cools to about 170° F., dissolve the sugar or honey in the water.

When it cools to about 70° F., add the *freshly* squeezed or just opened frozen juice, without bothering to dilute it. Just figure out how much of the frozen concentrate is needed to make the amount of diluted quantity called for in the recipe.

Add the yeast immediately and stir vigorously with a sterilized spoon, and cover. (1 pkg. bread yeast or 1 pkg. wine yeast)

As soon as the ferment has started, which should be in a day or two, add the flowers. Several times a day stir the flowers under with a sterilized spoon to keep them from drying out and inviting the dreaded vinegar bacteria.

No more than one week later, remove the flowers with the same sterilized spoon, pressing them with another sterilized spoon to squeeze out the precious wine in them.

Siphon the wine at this time into loosely stoppered large bottles. (Plastic wrap and a rubber band over the mouth of the bottle works well, or use a fermentation lock if you have it.) Store the wine in a cool place and bottle when clear, being careful to maintain complete cleanliness and boiling water sterility of all of your utensils and bottles. Don't pour wine, use a siphon.

Comments

An alternative method which insures greater destruction of the unwanted bacteria an
wild yeasts present in everything is to add all of the ingredients to the boiling water
however, a goodly amount of the more delicate fragrances depart with the steam. Th
addition of a tiny amount of potassium metabisulfite (1/10 t. per gallon) or a campde
tablet (sold in wine stores) to the first procedure before adding the yeast, will ki
unwanted microlife, and when the *wine* yeast is added *24 hours later* it will have
clean must to work on. A century of usage of this sulfur compound has bred yeast
able to live in low concentrations of this antiseptic. In twenty-four hours the SO
released from the potassium metabisulfite or campden tablet will have dissipate
somewhat.

If you use honey the wine will have a *distinctive* mead taste and be slightly heavy i
the head. White sugar which is sucrose is enzymatically transformed by the cleve
yeast into fructose and glucose. Fructose and glucose are the sugars in honey an
fruit. If you want an extra dose of B-vitamins to ease overindulgence, add a teaspoo
of "marmite," a vegetable concentrate sold in supermarkets.

Marigold wine is for serious connoisseurs of a good high. It takes three years to b
magical and delicious. If you can't wait that long, substitute about one quart of crushe
ripe crabapples for the marigolds and get a good party summer afternoon high i
about eight months.

—Contributed by Paul Fuge

COMPOUND BALM-WATER, COMMONLY CALLED EAU DE CARMES

TAKE of the fresh Leaves of Balm a quarter of a pound; Yellow Rind of
Lemons, two ounces; Nutmegs and Coriander seeds, of each one ounce;
Cloves, Cinnamon, and Angelica Root, of each half an ounce: having
pounded the spices and seeds and bruised the leaves and roots, put them
with a quart of Brandy into a glafs cucurbit, of which ftop the mouth, and
set it in a warm place, where let it remain two or three days. Then add a
pint of simple Balm-water, and shake the whole well together; after which
distill in a vapour bath till the ingredients are left almost dry; and preserve
the water thus obtained, in bottles well stopped.

This water has been long famous at Paris and London, and carried
thence to moft parts of Europe. It has the reputation of being a cordial of
very extraordinary virtues, and not only of availing in all lownefs of fpirits,
but even in apoplexies. It is alfo much efteemed in the cafes of the gont
in the ftomach; whence the Carmelite Friars, who originally were in
possession of the fecret, have reaped great benefit from the fale of this
water.

—The Toilet of Flora, 1779

Eau de Carmes is still for sale at Caswell-Massey in New York (See Chapter 7). They call it *Eau de Melisse des Carmes* and it is used for uneasy stomachs due to overeating, hangover, chills, etc.

HERB DRINKS

These herb drinks feature Chlorella, a very special unicellular organism that can probably provide the world with all the nutritive factors that it needs to survive in a healthy, happy state. Chlorella is a very high energy food that you can take in drinks or in capsule form. (See Chapter 6 for a mail-order address in California.)

FRUITEE-TOOTEE

8 oz. Apple juice
1 Banana

1 medium Apple or fruit of your choice
4 400 mg. capsules Chlorella
1 T. honey or rice syrup

Mix in a blender and drink. You can also add 2 T. trail mix (nuts, seeds, fruits) and 1 T. brewer's yeast to the blend.

CARACOCO ZAPA

8 oz. Carrot juice

4 oz. Coconut milk
3 400 mg. capsules Chlorella

Blend well in a blender.

Contributed by Tom Hart.

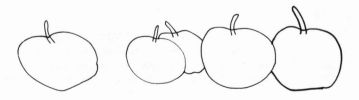

HERB JELLIES

Herb jelly on meat, toast or crackers, or poultry is a pleasant change from what you might be used to. It is easy to make and requires very little time or energy. Currently I have 4 different flower jellies in my refrigerator, and 3 other types to be used on meat and poultry. I must admit that I no longer make my own jellies or tracklements but purchase them from Truc International in Massachusetts (see Chapter 6).

MINT JELLY:

Boil chopped, tart, unpeeled Apples with water, and strain through a jelly bag to make Apple juice. To 1 pint of the Apple juice add 2 T. of white wine vinegar, the rind and juice of 1 Lemon, and 1 lb. of sugar. Heat this to boiling, stirring to dissolve the sugar. Drop in a large bunch of clean, stripped Mint stalks (the leaves having been removed), and boil for 5 minutes. Crush the Mint leaves, add them to the pot, and bring it to a boil again. Remove from the heat and take out the Mint stalks. Strain the liquid and pour it into sterilized jars. A fresh and clean Mint leaf and small Peppermint Geranium leaf can be added to each jar before sealing.

HERB JELLY:

Herb jelly can be made with any leaf or flower by following the basic recipe above and substituting the herb of your choice for the Mint. The basic formula is an Apple juice jelly, gelled with Lemon pectin.

FLOWER JELLY:

Flower jelly can also be made. (I am rather fond of Orange Petal jelly and Violet jelly.) Make an Apple juice jelly and gel it with Lemon Pectin. Cook it with some of the fresh flowers of your choice. Strain it and add more fresh and clean flowers to each jar before sealing.

HERB BUTTERS

Herb butters are simply herbs chopped finely and blended into sweet (unsalted) butter by mixing thoroughly and refrigerating it. These butters are delicious on vegetables, or as a spread for toast or crackers. They have not been widely used since Victorian times and have simply dropped out of fashion, possibly because herbs are not commonly grown these days. In most cases fresh herbs are preferable to dried herbs. But certainly dried herbs will do, such as Parsley or Chives, and of course carefully mashed seeds of one sort and another.

First buy top quality sweet butter, margarine will *not* do, and cream it with a fork or back of a wooden spoon. *Finely chop* fresh herbs, or powder by hand dried herbs (rub them briskly between your palms), and with a fork mash the herbs into the creamed butter (2 T. or more for each quarter-pound stick). Add just a touch of Lemon juice or white wine vinegar to bring up the flavor of the herbs, and refrigerate overnight to allow full flavor to develop.

Sage butter is good used over a roasting chicken. Tarragon butter goes well with meat or fish. Chervil-Parsley butter is excellent with vegetables. Spearmint or Dill butter is yummy with lamb chops. Fennel Leaf butter is a natural served with fish. Oregano butter is an excellent topping over green noodles (fettucine verde). And there is nothing more satisfying than Garlic butter on a crusty loaf of French bread.

FLOWER BUTTERS

In a wide-mouth enamel bowl alternate layers of soft, sweet butter and freshly picked, clean, dry flowers. Cover it tightly and set aside in a cool place so that the fragrance of the flowers permeates the butter.

You may use this method with Orange Flowers, Lemon Flowers, Borage Flowers, Lavendar Flowers, Honeysuckle Flowers, Jasmine Flowers, Mullein Flowers, and with any small, scented flower. Each flower has a different flavor, and so it will take time and practice to know which Flower Butter will go well in which dish. For examples: Lemon Flower Butter would be nice in a sweet icing as well as served on fish, and Borage Flower butter would be pleasing on crackers and served with a Cucumber salad.

HERB VINEGARS

I will not give individual recipes for herbal vinegars because they are all handled in the same way.

Gather fresh herbs and bruise them gently to release their volatile oils. Put them loosely into a clean, vinegar type of bottle, or even a pottery jar, filling the container loosely with the herbs. Add enough white or Apple cider vinegar, or even white wine vinegar, to fill the container. Cap it or seal with paraffin, and store in a warm, dry place for ten days or two weeks. At the end of this time, strain the vinegar into sterilized bottles, *label it,* put a fresh sprig of the herb into each bottle, seal or cork, and put away for use. Certain herbs, such as the Mediterranean type herbs (Oregano, Sage, Garlic, or Tarragon), can be made with red wine vinegar, as their taste and scent is strong enough to "come through" the vinegar. Vinegars can be made with mixtures of herbs, such as Garlic, Lemon Peel, and Mint, or Burnet and Borage Blossom, or Spearmint and Apple Mint. But, the vinegars work especially well with single herbs, such as Basil, Burnet, Chervil, Chive, Dill Seed, Garlic, Marjoram, Oregano, Parsley, Savory (both winter and summer types), Sage, Tarragon, or Thyme. You can also add Violet flowers to white vinegars to give an especially tangy taste and great color.

And what is "mother of vinegar," you ask? The "mother" is the rather slimy membrane that is formed at the bottom of the vinegar as it ferments; it is composed of bacteria and yeast. The "mother" of any particular kind of vinegar will hold true, and can be used when you make new vinegar to retain the true taste. This is why some "mothers" are handed down from generation to generation of vinegar makers to retain the fine old flavor. Add "mother" to any red or white wine that has been left standing open for a while and vinegar will be made in four to five weeks.

DISTILLED LAVENDAR VINEGAR

Put into a stone cucurbit any quantity of fresh gathered Lavendar Flowers picked clean from the Stalks; pour on them as much distilled Vinegar as is required to make the Flowers float; distill in a vapour bath, and draw off about three-fourths of the Vinegar.

In the same manner are prepared the Vinegars, all from all other vegetable substances. Compound Vinegars are made by mixing several aromatic substances together; observing only to bruise all hard woody ingredients, and to let them infuse a sufficient time in the Vinegar before you proceed to distillation.

Lavender Vinegar is of use for the Toilet; it is cooling, and when applied to the face, braces up the relaxed fibres of the skin.

—*The Toilet of Flora,* 1779

HERB MUSTARD

Mustards are useful when making salad dressings, particularly French or Italian oil and vinegar dressings. Herb mustards are also good on meats, hot dogs, vegetables, and as a spread for sandwiches or such things as pirochkis.

MUSTARD MUSTARD

2 T. or more dry Mustard seed ground to a powder and thinned with enough water to

work it into a thick paste. Add enough white wine, cream, vinegar or herb vinegar, depending on the flavor you desire, to give the paste the consistency of a thick cream. Mix in 2 t. of honey or sugar. Add salt and Pepper to taste. Add 1/4 t. Turmeric and 1 t. oil. Mix together and bottle for use.

TARRAGON MUSTARD

Follow the above directions, using the following proportions:

3 T. dry Mustard seed	1/4 t. Chile
1-1/2 t. Tarragon vinegar	pinch of pepper
1/4 t. Allspice	1/2 t. honey
	1 t. Tarragon oil, Olive oil or Red oil

DIJON MUSTARD is made with black Mustard seeds, water, vinegar and salt.

RUSSIAN MUSTARD is made with Mustard seeds, vinegar, sugar, honey, salt and garlic.

HOT DOG MUSTARD is made with mild Mustard seeds, vinegar, water, salt and Turmeric.

HERB HONEY

Herb honeys are good as sweetening agents, in marinades, or simply for roasting meats and for use as a medicine.

TWO WAYS TO PREPARE HERB HONEY:

1) In a small enamel pot add a large bunch of herbs, hips or flowers, and enough honey (mild tasting, such as Clover) just to cover the plant. Simmer gently over low flame for 1 hour. Strain out the plant. Add a sprig of the freshly picked and clean plant to each jar and bottle the honey.

2) In a small enamel pot add a large bunch of herbs, hips or flowers, and enough water just to cover the plant. Simmer for 1 hour and strain through a ricer, chinois or cheesecloth. Add an equal quantity of honey to the liquid, return to the fire and cook gently until the liquid is reduced by a third.

ROSEHIP HONEY (for Waffles, Toast or for a Sore Throat):

Fill a quart jar with freshly picked Rose hips. Bring some water to a boil and pour the water over the hips. Cover and let this steep overnight. The hips should be mushy; if not, cook gently over low heat until they are. Press the hips and water through a coarse sieve or chinois. To the purée, add an equal amount of honey. Store in the refrigerator. Use as soon as possible.

SAGE HONEY:

Follow method #1 using freshly picked Sage tops and Sage Honey (nectar gathered by bees from sage blossoms, transformed alchemically by the bees into honey, and commercially called "Sage Honey"). Sage Honey is good for colds or respiratory problems where there is an excess amount of mucous.

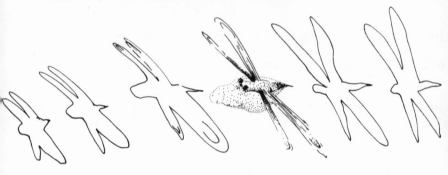

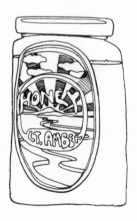

OTHER HERB STUFF & CONDIMENTS

To Pickle Nasturtium Buds. Gather your nasturtium seed pods quickly
after the Blossoms are off: put them in cold Water and Salt for three days,
move them about once a day; make a Pickle but do not boil of White
wine, White wine vinegar, Shallots, Pepper, Horseradish, Cloves, Salt,
and Mace whole and Nutmeg quartered; then put in your seeds and stop
them close; they are to be eaten as capers.

—Compleat Housewife,
London, 1739

SZECHUAN CONDIMENTS

Red oil and red vinegar are very versatile, on cold or hot noodles they are
delicious, and definitely recommended for a cold and a sore throat. Get Chinese
noodles, cook them according to directions, and refrigerate. When they are cold serve
the noodles with a bit of Cilantro. Add red oil and vinegar according to your fancy.

Boil up a chicken and skin it. Cut the meat into pieces. Add the Red oil and vinegar
to taste.

Add Red oil and vinegar on vegetables, noodles, cold meats, poultry or fish.

RED OIL:

Take a small bottle and fill it with hot dried red Chiles. Add 4 or 5 cloves of peeled
Garlic. Add 1 Star Anise seed. Fill the jar full of Peanut oil. Refrigerate bottle until
needed.

RED VINEGAR:

Take a small bottle and fill it full of hot, dried, red Chiles. Add 1 or 2 cloves of peeled
Garlic. Add 1 Star Anise seed. Fill the bottle full of Rice vinegar. Refrigerate bottle until
needed.

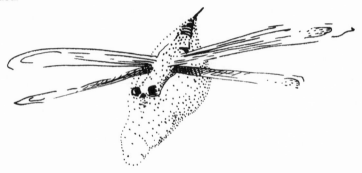

CANDIED ANGELICA STEMS

Before the Angelica flowers, cut its stems in pieces 2−4 inches long. Boil them until tender. Remove them from the water and cool until they can be handled, then peel the outer skin. Return the peeled stems to the water and boil them, uncovered, with some dark green Cabbage or Grape leaves until they become very green. Strain them, throw away the Cabbage or Grape leaves, and let the stems dry. Then weigh them. Allow 1 lb. of granulated sugar for every pound of Angelica stems. Spread the stems out in a shallow glass dish and sprinkle more sugar over them. Cover and leave them for several days so that the stems can absorb some of the sugar. Then boil the sugared stems very carefully, not letting the sugar burn. You may have to add a bit of liquid here. When they are boiling well, take the pan off the fire, remove the Angelica from the pan, and add up to 1/2 cup more granulated sugar to the syrup in the pan. Heat this syrup until the sugar dissolves, place the Angelica back in the pan, and boil again for 3−5 minutes. Again remove the pan from the fire and let it cool until you can remove the Angelica stems. Place the stems on plates, and put the plates into a very cool oven (225°) until the stems are quite dry. Cool them. Store them in airtight jars.

Variations of this recipe can be found in *A Modern Herbal,* p. 39, and *Herbs with Everything,* p. 12. For other recipes for candied Angelica, please check *A Modern Herbal.*

Part III

The Secrets

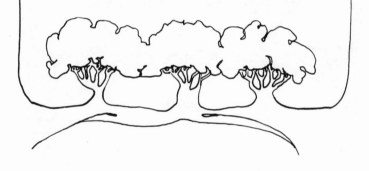

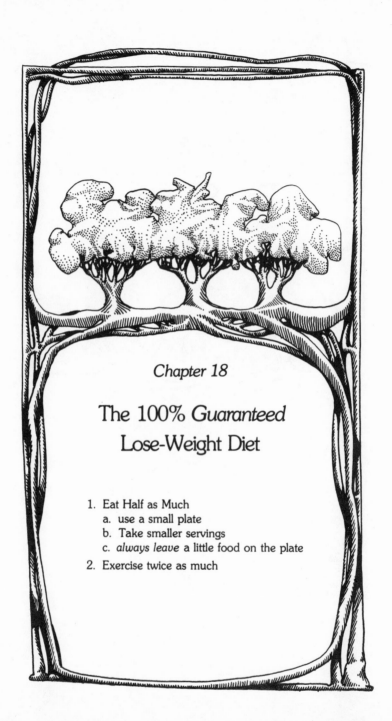

Chapter 18

The 100% Guaranteed
Lose-Weight Diet

1. Eat Half as Much
   a. use a small plate
   b. Take smaller servings
   c. *always leave* a little food on the plate
2. Exercise twice as much

Chapter 19

Cooking Magic

RICE COOKED IN EIGHT PRECIOUS SHADOWS

This dish is supposed to inspire delightful dreams, but you must not dream of anything that has to do with eating or you will wake up to sorrow.

1 lb. Rice	Some Jujube fruit, chopped
3–4 C. water plus about 1 C. more added later	2 oz. crushed Ginger root
	Some pitted Cherries, chopped
Peanut oil	Some pitted Dates, chopped
1/2 C. or more sugar	Some candied Oranges, chopped
Bit of Lotus flower, chopped	Some pitted Plums, chopped
1/2 oz. Lychi, chopped	A few pieces crushed Cinnamon

Thoroughly wash the rice, preferably soaking it overnight. Cook it covered in 3–4 C. water in a heavy iron pan until the Rice is opaque in the middle but not soft. Add more water, about 1 C., some Peanut oil, and the sugar. Bring to a boil, reduce heat and cook 15 minutes more.

Make a mixture of the remaining ingredients. Divide this mixture into 8 parts, place each part in a buttered porcelain cup (coddling egg cup or individual ramekin) and add a little of the cooked rice on top of each cup.

Place the cups in a saucepan that is half-filled with rice, and place the saucepan on a rack in a covered steaming pot half-filled with water. Cook until the pot is dry. Surround with water again and cook until the saucepan is almost dry (about 3 hours). Serve hot. The rice should be quite tender and the pudding firm.

Serves 8.

TO ENABLE ONE TO SEE THE FAIRIES

Take 1 pint of virgin olive oil and wash it with rosewater and marigold water until it is white. The Roses and the Marigolds are to be gathered towards the east and the water thereof to be made of pure spring water. Put the washed oil into a vial glass and add Hollyhock buds, Marigold flowers, wild Thyme tops and flowers, young Hazel buds, and the grass of a faery throne. The Thyme must be gathered near the side of a hill where fairies used to be. Set the glass in the sun for three days so that the ingredients can become incorporated. Then put away for use.

—Formula dated 1600

Mrs. Kathleen Bennett of Pottstown, Pa. saw this formula in my book, *Herbs & Things,* and added this note. "To use the formula, one should annoint the eyes and just go about one's daily business. As a word of caution, *always* wear something iron on your body while the formula is working to avert the power of the Faerie. If this is not done the person working the formula may either 'be taken' or blinded by those he may chance to see." In a later letter Mrs. Bennett says, "Irish oral tradition is full of accounts of individuals who are suddenly capable of seeing the faerie against the will of the faerie. These involve the splashing or touching of water that has touched a faerie or rarely, a potion, all of which are applied to the eyes. One never has to sit around and wait. The Faeries are not so many 'Tinkerbells' flittering on buttercups and scattering stardust. Legends about them are many. Some are called 'Tuotha del Danaan' and are believed to have been an early Celtic race. All in all, they are a people of some previous age: tall, beautiful and majestic, and they are invisible to ordinary humans unless they grant sight or it is accidentally obtained. The 'Tuatha del Danaan' are said to walk and live as you or I and that a human with sight may meet a faerie anywhere. There is, of course, a catch, and that is that the faerie can put one or both of the persons eyes out. It is sad though, that being from another age their power is useless over Iron (I should think steel also). Therefore one should wear something iron when venturing among them.

These things seem to only apply to the land faerie, the silkies, mellowmen, etc. appear and disappear and although they don't take offense at being seen they often 'take' people."

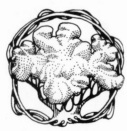

MAGICAL FOODS

Agrimony has been used in magic to heal the eyes and when put under a man's head so that he would sleep as if dead.

> "If it be laid under a man's head,
> He shall sleep as he were dead;
> He shall never dread be waken
> Till from under his head it be taken."

Agrimony flower spikes, when mixed with Mugwort and infused in apple cider vinegar, and eaten regularly as the acid in a salad dressing, is said in time to remove warts, and cure a bad back.

Borage, according to Pliny: Use the flowers in salads to exhilarate and make the mind glad. Borage blossoms drive away sadness and increase joy. The tender parts of the plant infused in wine make men and women glad and drive away dullness. A syrup made of Borage flowers is used to comfort the heart and quiet a frantic and lunatical person. The leaves, especially raw in salad, give good blood, especially to those who have been recently sick. And of course Borage steeped in wine is identical with the famous Nepenthe, and brought absolute forgetfulness. We even find Borage of use to students to cheer them up and help their mental faculties, and to revive the hypochondriac.

For Melancholia, Pluck petals from the lovely red Rose, pick fresh Violets, and Borage too, dry them in the warm sun, mix them lovingly together, and seal them up carefully so that they will not lose their savor. When you are depressed and sad and your life seems not right, take a small handful of the dried flowers and put them into your best teapot. Carefully pour over the flowers about 2 cups of boiling water. Add a dollop of Rosemary honey and infuse for 5 minutes in the sun. Sit in the sun with a lovely teacup and fill it full of the Flower tea; drink slowly as much as you like. Your sadness will soon melt away.

Marshmallow Root Ointment rubbed on the body is said to cure those who have been cursed by witchcraft, and is especially good to protect a body against hot metals. If you make old-fashioned Marshmallow Root Marshmallows and eat them, this is also said to protect the eater against all manner of hot things. (To make Marshmallows make a decoction of Marshmallow root, gel it with gelatin, Irish moss or Gum Arabic, sweeten with sugar, let it solidify in a buttered pan, cut into squares, and roll each square in powdered sugar. Store in an airtight jar and eat when needed.)

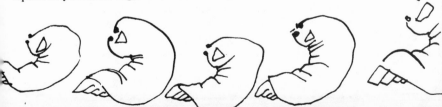

Orchid roots were once thought to be the food of the satyrs, and thus they developed not only a magical reputation, but also an aphrodisiacal one. William Coles said, "The full and plump Roots of the Orchid are efficacious to provoke one to Lust, when they are full they do by Signature but if they are skinny and lean they will mortify lust. That here is a remedy that helps Nature if it is deficient and restrains it if it is too luxuriant . . ."

An Orchid gel can be made by taking some powdered roots and boiling them in 2 cups of water. When it begins to gel, add some wine, some sugar, some Vanilla oil (2 drops), and some Lemon juice. Mix it up and set aside for later use.

Rooibosch Wine, if frequently consumed, will relieve arthritis and rheumatism. Take 2 handfuls of the herb, one handful of raisins, one handful of good hops, 10 quarts of water; boil it up for some time, strain it and then add 1 cake of active yeast and sugar to taste. Boil this for 10 more minutes, bottle it in sterile bottles, and let it stand for 2 days. When fermentation is complete, seal the bottles and let the wine age for 6 months before using. The medicinal value of this wine is not due to the hops contained.

Rue, when added to condiments, is a remedy for nervous indigestion, especially that which occurs when eating before strangers, which of course is the result of witchcraft.

EGYPTIAN LOVE POTION

Take by the light of the full moon; the potion will infuse your glands and enrich the blood.

—found on an Egyptian papyrus

1 pint of water
1 oz. mashed Licorice root

1 oz. sesame seed, mashed
1 oz. bruised Fennel seed
honey

Place all ingredients in a pot and bring to a boil. Reduce to simmer and simmer for 5 minutes. Turn off heat and infuse until cold. Strain. Take 1/2 oz. twice a day, with your lover's hair wrapped about your fingers, while intoning the magic ritualistic words:

I am possessed by burning love for this man whose name is
_____ and whose lock of hair I hold in my hand. Let the man yearn for me, desire me, let his desire burn for me! Let this love come forth from the spirit, and enter him. Magnetize the potion with his love-force. I love him, want him: I drink this potion (drink half and later he drinks other half) and my desire reaches out to him. Oh Gods, let him become filled with love. O spirits of the air search him out and fill him with the winds of love. Oh Gods of the brink let him burn with love for me.

—A very old formula

Bibliography

A bibliography is a map that the reader can use to follow the progression of the author's research, thereby showing how the author arrived at the conclusions and knowledge conveyed in the body of the work. These books listed are the ones that seemed most important to me. Since my recipes are inherited and I have literally thousands of recipes collected over the last thirty years and over one hundred cookbooks that made interesting reading, it then seemed only natural that only the cookbooks that I have actually enjoyed and seem to me to be originals in their field are listed. Most recipes are just repeats from one book to another. The books starred are those that seem to be particularly useful in a work of this sort. And if you pursue my bibliographical path, then you will indeed see how I arrived at some rather bizarre positions in the field of herbalism.

Allen, Gayle and Robert Fletcher. *The Egg Book*. Millbrae, Ca.: Celestial Arts, 1975.

*Bianchini, Francesco. *The Complete Book of Fruits & Vegetables*. New York: Crown Publishers, 1973.

*_____ *Health Plants of the World*. New York: Newsweek Books, 1977.

Boxer, Arabella. *Nature's Harvest, The Vegetable Cookbook*. Chicago: Henry Regnery Co., 1974.

*Bryan, John E. *The Edible Ornamental Garden*. San Francisco: 101 Productions, 1974.

Calella, Organic John. *Let There Be Food*. Berkeley, Ca.: And/Or Press.

Carcione, Joe. *The Green Grocer*. New York: Pyramid Books, 1974.

Claire, Rosine. *French Gourmet Vegetarian Cookbook*. Millbrae, Ca.: Celestial Arts, 1975.

*Culpeper, Nicholas. *Culpeper's English Physician: And Complete English Physician . . . Family Dispensatory*. 15th edition. London: W. Lewis, M.DCCC.XIII.

Darby, William J. *Food: The Gift of Osiris*. 2 volumes. New York: Academic Press, 1977.

*Delfs, Robert A. *The Good Food of Szechwan*. New York: Kodansha International, 1974.

*de Sounin, Leonie. *Magic in Herbs*. New York: M. Barrows & Co., 1941. This is truly a delightful work, full of the love and care the author lavishes on her foods and plants. I highly recommend it.

Digbie, Sir Kenelme. *The Closet of the Eminently Learned Sir Kenelme Digbie Kt. Opened: . . . Published by his Son's Confent*. London: Printed by E. C. for H. Brome, 1669.

Gabriel, Ingred. *Herb Identifier and Handbook.* New York: Sterling Publishing Co., 1970.

Gerarde, John. *The Herball or Generall Hiftorie of Plantes.* Volumes I, II. London: Printed by Adam Norton and Richard Whitakers, 1636.

*Geuter, Maria. *Herbs in Nutrition.* London: Bio-Dyamil Agric. Assn., 1962.
This is most definitely a must book in the field of nutrition and herbs.

Gordon, Jean. *The Art of Cooking with Roses.* New York: Noonday Press, 1968.

*Grieve, Mrs. M. *A Modern Herbal.* 2 volumes. New York: Hafner Publishing Co., 1931.
A must work for the beginning herbalist.

————. Culinary Herbs and Condiments. New York: Harcourt, Brace and Co., 1934.

Hanle, Zack. *Cooking with Flowers.* Los Angeles: Price/Stern/Sloan, 1971.

Harris, Ben Charles. *Better Health with Culinary Herbs.* Barre, Mass.: Barre Publ., 1952.

Harris, Lloyd J. *The Book of Garlic.* San Francisco: Panjandrum Press, 1974.
A terrific book about Garlic that contains the only known photograph of the pregnant Jeanne Rose.

Hortus Third. Staff of the L. H. Bailey Hortorium, Cornell University. New York: Macmillan Co., 1976.

*Howard, Sheila. *Herbs with Everything.* New York: Holt, Rinehart and Winston, 1976.
This is really a fine work, with lovely illustrations.

*Kennedy, Diana. *The Tortilla Book.* New York: Harper & Row, 1975.

Kimball, Yeffe and Jean Anderson. *The Art of American Indian Cooking.* Garden City, N.Y.: Doubleday & Co., 1965.

Kirschmann, John. *Nutrition Almanac.* New York: McGraw-Hill, 1973.

*Leyel, Mrs. C. F. *Cinquefoil.* London: Faber and Faber, 1957.

————. *Cold Savoury Meals.* London: George Routledge & Sons, Ltd., 1927.

Li, Shih-Chen. *Chinese Medicinal Herbs (Pen Ts'ao).* San Francisco: Georgetown Press, 1973.

Loewenfeld, Claire and Phillippa Back. *The Complete Book of Herbs and Spices.* New York: G. P. Putnam's Sons, 1974.

Los Angeles Times. Waverly Root's many articles on herbs and foods.
If you are interested in herbs and foods, get Waverly Root's many articles published in the *L.A. Times.*

MacNichol, Mary. *Flowery Cookery.* New York: Collier Books, 1974. This is a wonderfully done book.

Miller, Joseph. *Botanicum Officinale; Or a Compendious Herbal.* London: Printed for E. Bell in Cornhill, M.DCC.XXII.

Millspaugh, Charles F. *American Medicinal Plants.* New York: Dover Publ., 1974. Original printing date 1892.

Neruda, Pablo. *Selected Poems of Pablo Neruda.* A bilingual edition edited and translated by Ben Belitt. New York: Grove Press, 1961.

*Niethammer, Carolyn. *American Indian Food and Lore.* New York: Collier Books, 1974.
This is a wonderfully done book.

*Nilson, Bee. *Herb Cookery.* New York: Hippocrene Books, 1974. A truly interesting and useful herb cookery book. Much information.

Parkinson, John. *Paradisi in Sole Paradisus Terrestris*. London: Methuen & Co., 1629.
    Faithfully reprinted from the edition of 1629.

*Pliny, the Elder. *Pliny's Natural History*. Translated by Philemon Holland. London: 1601.

Rohde, Eleanour Sinclair. *Rose Recipes*. London: George Routledge & Sons, Ltd., 1939.

_____. *Uncommon Vegetables*. London: Country Life, Ltd., 1943.

Rombauer, Irma S. *The Joy of Cooking*. New York: Bobbs-Merrill Co., 1931.

*Rose, Jeanne. *Herbs & Things*. New York: Grosset & Dunlap, 1972. An herbal primer.

_____. *The Herbal Body Book*. New York: Grosset & Dunlap, 1976.
    An herbal body care book.

_____ *Kitchen Cosmetics*. San Francisco: Panjandrum Press, 1977.

Rutherford, Meg. *A Pattern of Herbs*. New York: Dolphin Books, 1976. A wonderful book;
    herbs for goodness, food and health, beautifully illustrated but greatly marred by the lack of
    an index.

*Schery, Robert W. *Plants for Man*. 2nd edition. New York: Prentice-Hall, 1972.

Silverman, Maida. *A City Herbal*. New York: Alfred A. Knopf, 1977.

Simmons, Paula. *The Zucchini Cookbook*. Seattle: Pacific Search, 1974.

Skinner, Charles M. *Myths and Legends of Flowers, Trees, Fruits, and Plants*. London: J. B.
    Lippincott Co., 1913.
    My copy of this wonderful book originally belonged to Louise Beebe Wilder, author of The
    Fragrant Path.

Tannahill, Reay. *Food in History*. New York: Stein and Day, 1973.

The Toilet of Flora; Or a Collection of the Most Simple and Approved Methods of Preparing . . .
    Reprinted from the edition dated 1779. London: J. Murray.

van der Veer, Katherine. *Herbs for Urbans and Suburbans*. New York: Loker Raley, 1938.

Wilson, Jose and Arthur Leaman. *The Complete Food Catalogue*. New York: Holt, Rinehart
    and Winston, 1977.

Zane, Eva. *Middle Eastern Cookery*. San Francisco: 101 Productions, 1974.

Zelayeta, Elena. *Elena's Secrets of Mexican Cooking*. Garden City, N.Y.: Doubleday & Co.,
    1958.

The following books or magazines are continually producing recipes of continuing interest. Get a
subscription.

Composition and Facts about Foods. Ford Heritage. Woodstown, N.J.

Gourmet Magazine. 777 3rd Ave., New York, N.Y.

The Herbal Review. 34 Boscobel Pl. London SW 1, England.

The Herbarist. (A publication of the Herb Society of America) 300 Massachusetts Ave., Boston,
    Mass.

*Lovers of the Stinking Rose. (An organization devoted to the glorification of Garlic; their
    publication is called *The Garlic Times*.) 1043 Cragmont Ave., Berkeley, Ca.

Prevention Magazine. Emmaus Pa. 18049.

Well-being Magazine. 833 W. Fir. San Diego, Ca. 92101.

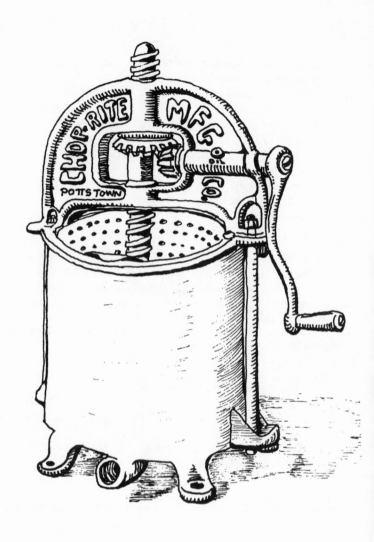

Index of Recipes

JEANNE ROSE'S HERBAL GUIDE TO INNER HEALTH INDEX

NOTE: Page numbers in *italic* type refer to the Materia Medica chapter.
Page numbers in **boldface** type refer to actual recipes.

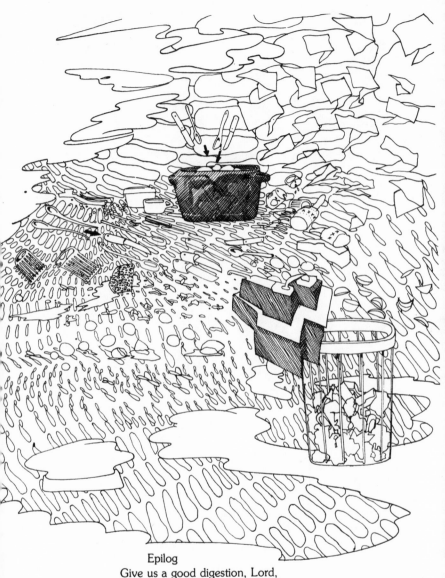

Epilog

Give us a good digestion, Lord,
And also something to digest.
Give us a healthy body, Lord,
With sense to keep it at its best,

Give us a sense of humor, Lord,
Give us the grace to see a joke,
To get some happiness from life,
And pass it on to other folk. Amen.

Found in Chester Cathedral, Chester,
England, 18th century